Michael van Straten is Britain's leading holistic practitioner. A practising and registered osteopath, naturopath and accupuncturist, he practises from his clinic in London W1. He also writes freelance for all the major newspapers and magazines and broadcasts regularly on cable television and radio reaching millions of people every week with his unique brand of helpful, cheerful advice on complementary medicine.

He is the author, with Barbara Griggs, of the bestselling *Superfoods* and *The Superfoods Diet Book* and his book *The New Body Talk* was recently reissued by Headline.

Jacky Fleming is a bestselling cartoonist. Her books, *Be a Bloody Train Driver*, *Never Give Up* and *Falling in Love* are published by Penguin.

Line drawings by **Noel Chamberlain**.

BACK TO STRENGTH

Self help for back pain

Michael van Straten

HEADLINE

First published in 1994
by Headline Book Publishing

10 9 8 7 6 5 4 3 2 1

ISBN 0 7472 4381 6

Typeset by
Letterpart Limited, Reigate, Surrey

Printed and bound in Great Britain by
HarperCollins Manufacturing, Glasgow

HEADLINE BOOK PUBLISHING
A division of Hodder Headline PLC
338 Euston Road
London NW1 3BH

DEDICATION

This book is dedicated to my alma mater, the British College of Naturopathy and Osteopathy, and the pioneering spirits who founded it. Without them, I and hundreds like me would never have been osteopaths. It is also dedicated to all the patients who have seen fit to put their backs in my hands during the past thirty-five years, in the profound hope that reading it will keep them and others out of my hands in the future.

ACKNOWLEDGEMENTS

I am grateful to the invaluable assistance of David O'Neill, the Librarian at the Anglo-European College of Chiropractic, to the Principal, Professor Brian Kliger, and to J.M. Langworthy of the Research Department. Between them they provideed a vast amount of highly specialised research material which I would not have had access to without their help and enthusiasm.

This book would not have seen the light of day without Janet Betley's constant spur and frequent burning of the midnight oil. She has not only typed every word but also saved me from endless disasters with the computer. She has spent far too many hours without rest at the keyboard, which will no doubt result in a chronic back complaint, but she types on in uncomplaining silence. I must also thank her husband Tony and her daughters Louise and Kathy who have spent many boring hours sitting in my house while mother slaved away.

Contents

Introduction

It's thirty-five years since I decided to become an osteo-path rather than a doctor. My medical friends were horrified and said I'd spend the rest of my life dealing with the work-shy masses suffering from that well-known disease, classified by doctors as 'plumbus oscillandi' – swinging the lead. Because you couldn't see a backache, the perceived wisdom was that it was the greatest excuse of all time for skiving off work and being a layabout. I can honestly say that thirty-five years later I would not need the fingers of both hands to count the number of lead-swingers that I've seen.

It wasn't just my medical friends who were horrified – I didn't dare tell my parents either, not that is until I rescued my father from six weeks in hospital in a plaster cast, took him home, cut off the plaster and finally confessed. Osteopathic treatment soon had him back on his feet. He'd never been in hospital before, and I'm happy to say has never been there since.

Back pain is so common that if you've never had it, the chances are that your turn is not far away. Four out of five people will suffer from it at some time in their lives. The scale of the problem is huge and its total cost is impossible to calculate both in economic and social terms. Look at the following statistics:

- At least 67 million certified working days are lost through back pain every year in the UK and that's not

counting pensioners and members of the armed forces.
- 80 per cent of people who have one attack of backache get another.
- There are 2.25 million visits to GPs for back problems each year.
- 1.5 million people are on invalidity benefit due to back-related conditions.
- 10 per cent of the 63,000 people hospitalised with backache have surgery.
- Hospitalisation and surgery for back problems cost the NHS £350 million per annum.
- 500,000 people suffer work-related backache every year.
- 3,600 nurses leave the NHS each year through backache.
- It costs the NHS £120 million a year in nurse absence and replacement due to backache.
- 80 per cent of all VDU workers will suffer backache.
- Working drivers are three times more likely to suffer.
- Sedentary workers are just as likely to get backache as manual workers.

These figures from the National Back Pain Association tell us about the scale of the problem. What they don't tell us is the devastating effect that backache has on individuals and families – how many fathers can't kick a football around the garden with their children; how many mothers find pushing a vacuum cleaner too painful to bear; how many couples give up on sex because one or other and sometimes both are in too much pain.

In spite of these staggering figures controversy rages over the value of the wide variety of available treatments – surgery, traction and corsets, plaster casts, exercise, rest, physiotherapy, injections, drugs, acupuncture, chiropractic and osteopathy – every practitioner thinks their therapy is the answer and every sufferer thinks their own personal expert is the best in the world. The truth is that it's horses for courses. I see patients who swear that the last practitioner they consulted was nothing but a charlatan when I know that they were probably one of the best people in their field in the world. I'm also certain that patients who I have failed to 'cure' say that they wouldn't recommend me to their worst enemy – not even their bank manager!

Men and women with back pain just want to get on with their lives. They are desperate to go back to work, back to their sporting or leisure activities, back to having fun with their children or grandchildren and maybe just back to the corner shop for their morning paper. Back pain is frustrating and depressing because it interferes with almost every activity from washing your hair to driving your car, earning your living, having a bath and even enjoying a normal and active sex life.

Sex is the one aspect of back pain which is seldom mentioned in the many text books and those written for the lay public. Any practical advice for the unfortunate couple who have abandoned the joys of sex because no one will help them overcome the pain and discomfort would stick out like a sore thumb. It just isn't there. Even the patients that I see are reluctant to bring up the subject; it usually requires a leading question or two to establish that their partner is getting fed up with the deprivation. The real fear, of course, is that they will look elsewhere!

There is much discussion of the psychosomatic or 'malingerer's' back. It is a fact that some patients do fall into this category and use the backache as an excuse to avoid intercourse as well as work, but the number is a tiny percentage of the millions of true sufferers from back pain. The experienced practitioner can soon identify the real case of lead-swinging and can refer those people for the appropriate treatment since, even if not caused by a physical problem, their pain and disability are very real to them.

I hope that this book will be of practical value and that it will encourage individuals to help themselves to a better back, to talk about their sexual problems with their practitioners, and, even more importantly, with each other. Your partner is unlikely to be psychic, and your continued and unexplained refusals will create a fearful aura of doubt, mistrust and frustration, and will often lead to the divorce court. Likewise your employer, school or university should be kept fully informed as they are not psychic either. With the right help and encouragement you can beat the back brat at his own game. Man or woman, adult or child, parent or grandparent – you must never give up. Instead, be brave, persevere with your chosen course of treatment, exercise, practise preventive back care and follow the path that will lead eventually, hopefully, happily but not always painlessly back to work, back to play, back to sex and best of all – back to strength.

CHAPTER 1

A Little Knowledge
is a Disaster

Each year thousands of patients parade their bad backs
through my consulting rooms and they nearly all have
two things in common – FEAR and IGNORANCE. Fear
for their future, since their minds are filled with old
wives' tales, half truths, and misunderstood information from other practitioners, to say nothing of the
mental picture of the wheelchair in which they confidently expect to end their days. Ignorance of even the
most basic knowledge of their own bodies and the spine
in particular. For some strange reason the spine has
become imbued with almost as much mystique as the
soul and the osteopath now possesses the legendary
powers of Merlin.

There is nothing magic or mystical about your back or
the right treatment for your pain. The spine is a mechanical structure and the osteopath a good mechanic. If your
lawnmower breaks down, you don't panic, you get it put
right and you certainly don't pamper it when it's fixed,
you still use it to cut the grass. You can even learn to take
care of it yourself. Your back is no different from the
lawnmower – you can get it fixed; you can enjoy a normal
active life and you must learn to take care of it yourself.
Understanding the anatomy and mechanics of the spine is
the first step towards prevention of future problems, and
prevention is better than cure.

BACK FEARS AND MYTHS

Here are some of the most common things my patients say to me when they come into my consulting room.

I've got a slipped disc.

This mythical phenomenon does not exist – when you understand the anatomy of the spine you'll know why. The disc simply bulges on one side and can cause pressure on the spinal nerves and this causes pain. You think that it's your disc that hurts. Not so. The intervertebral disc has no sensory nerves and can feel nothing. Your disc CAUSES back pain but is not painful itself.

I've got backache so there must be something wrong with my spine.

Not necessarily so – many different and often seemingly trivial problems can cause pain in the back, particularly conditions of the feet, ankles, knees and hips, since these can alter your weight distribution and place uneven stress on the joints of your spine. It is essential to examine the back patient thoroughly and to observe him walking, sitting, standing and lying down *without* clothes on.

One 42-year-old man came to me in desperation. He had suffered chronic back pain for five months and had been prescribed all sorts of treatment – rest, exercises, pills and physiotherapy, all to no avail. X-rays showed nothing and his doctor had hinted darkly of 'more drastic measures'. When I asked him to strip to his underpants he showed some reluctance. 'It is quite painful to get my trousers on and off and impossible to get to my socks without help – the doctor felt my back through my shirt.' What a pity, since after helping with the socks I found a large, very painful verruca in the patient's left sole. The verruca was

6

removed, the patient's gait returned to normal and the back pain vanished. The only drastic measure employed was a local anaesthetic to the foot.

My doctor said my spine was degenerating. Does that mean I'll end up in a wheelchair?

Absolutely not. 'Degenerative changes' is just medical jargon for arthritis and most people have some degenerative change in their vertebrae caused by normal wear and tear. In fact, as you get older these changes can actually help. The over-sixties rarely suffer from mechanical back problems, as their spines become more rigid as the discs between the vertebrae get narrower and the back becomes more stable. In fact, many chronic back sufferers find that their condition improves as they get older.

Fear of the unknown is common in us all. Unfortunately many practitioners foster this fear in their patients by using medical terms which they understand, but patients don't, such as the following:

Sciatica Pain in the leg
Cervical spondylosis Something wrong with the joints of the neck
Lumbago Backache
Exaggerated kyphosis, lordosis or scoliosis Your posture is not as good as it might be.

Don't be intimidated, if you don't know exactly what the doctor means, ask. I know that the more the patient understands exactly what their problem is and the reasons for the course of treatment I propose, the more likely they are to cooperate with enthusiasm. Patients should see their X-rays, have explanations with drawings if appropriate, and, above all, ask as many questions as they like. This all takes time but it is without doubt time well

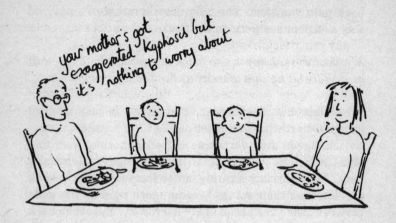

your mother's got exaggerated Kyphosis but it's nothing to worry about

spent, and will pay dividends later.

I've had trouble with my back for months, the doctor says I will need an operation.

No is the simple answer. Spinal surgery is the exception *not* the rule, and then only as a last resort for most people, though there are some cases in which early surgery is vital. Only 500 patients out of every 10,000 with back pain will see an orthopaedic surgeon, and only 25 of those are likely to have an operation. The decision to operate must only be taken after all other avenues of treatment have been thoroughly explored and all possible tests and investigations carried out.

When is surgery necessary?
It is a common misconception that all osteopaths are anti-surgery. The skilled manipulator who is properly trained in diagnosis will know when it is time to send his patient to see a surgeon, and the time to consider surgery is:

1. When repeated acute attacks are so frequent as to prevent work and disrupt normal social life.
2. When pain is severe, prolonged and does not respond to any other treatment.
3. When the patient is severely incapacitated.
4. If there is obvious muscle-wasting and paralysis.
5. When there is obvious nerve involvement and loss of bladder or bowel function. This situation calls for very early surgical intervention.

What will the surgeon do when operating on a painful back? He will either fix together two or more vertebrae so preventing movement of the joint which is causing pain or he will relieve pressure on the spinal nerve caused by a damaged disc, a bony spur or the narrowing of the space available for the nerve. Neither of these operations is a 'cure' for a bad back, but they can give relief from the symptoms. Long-term benefit depends on the patient's willingness to work on the 'holistic' approach to a strong, healthy spine, but more of this later.

I suppose I shall have to give up my job.

Unless you are a docker, coalman, professional weight-lifter or miner, the answer is most specifically NO. You will have to learn to do your job in a better way. Many back problems start with bad posture, and this causes stress on parts of the spine not designed to cope with extra weight-bearing. Sadly it is true that these postural faults are nearly always man-made. They start as early as primary school with unsuitable desks and chairs, and continue throughout life. Furniture in home and office, work benches in factories, car seats, machinery and even shoes and shoulder bags, can all contribute to your back-ache.

I am so often appalled at the shortsightedness and

meanness of employers, who complain endlessly of poor productivity, sickness and absenteeism and yet will not devote some time and money to improve the postural working conditions of their staff. Most firms spend fortunes on new technology in the office – electronic typewriters, word processors, VDUs, complex switchboards and the latest style of 'in' decor, but begrudge £200 for a good chair and footstool for the secretary who is responsible for these expensive new toys.

In hairdressing salons in every High Street, the potted palms and sophisticated sound systems take precedence over adjustable chairs. Domestic architects and property developers are no less to blame. Profit is the over-riding motive and economies are made by standardisation – but people are not standard. Do try to get the height of basins, cupboards, shelves and kitchen work tops that suits your build.

Some years ago I saw a 33-year-old man who was very fit and athletic but was considering giving up his job as a spare parts manager in a large garage. He always got severe backache at work. He thought this was due to lifting car parts and carrying them for his customers. Since few of the parts were heavy and his main sport was rugby, which did not affect his back – in fact he always felt better after the weekend – I was puzzled, so went to see him at work. The solution was obvious – he was 6'2" tall and spent a lot of time standing up writing out orders on a 2'6" high counter. We found an empty wooden crate, placed it upside down on top of the counter and that's where he now does his writing. Not only is his back pain cured without any treatment, but several of his taller colleagues also use his new 'desk' to advantage.

Some enlightened firms are now employing osteopaths to advise on postural matters. The rewards are very good, not only in financial terms for the employers, but more importantly, in few occurrences of back problems in the labour force.

My pain is always worse after sleeping, sitting or driving, what should I do?

Beds can produce real problems. Many couples are still sleeping in the same bed after 15 years of marriage, during which the car, fridge, cooker and furniture have seen several changes. Do not be conned by glossy adverts for orthopaedic beds designed by back specialists and costing hundreds of pounds. Your bed should be soft enough for comfort and to avoid pain on the pressure points of heels, hips, buttocks and shoulders, but firm enough underneath to avoid sagging. Any reputable bed manufacturer will supply you with an extra-firm mattress, but this is of little use if your base has soft edges and a dip in the middle. A bed board of 3/4" ply will provide enough support.

Make sure you test a new bed. Don't be too shy to lie on it for at least 10–15 minutes in the store. A really cheap and good bed is made of 3/4" or 1" ply with a number of 1" holes bored through it, supported on 8 bricks. This, with a mattress of 4" dense upholstery foam will suit most people.

If you travel a lot, ask hotels to provide a bed board, as most have them now. You can also buy a plastic folding board that will fit in the bottom of your suitcase. If all else fails, put the mattress on the floor. You may get some strange looks from the chambermaid, or your host, but that is better than being unable to get out of bed the next morning!

Chairs cause as many problems as beds for the back pain sufferer. Not only do they aggravate existing conditions, but bad seating is often a contributory factor. Modern furniture is often designed for looks not comfort. Sofas and armchairs tend to be far too soft, have seats which are too deep, backs which are too low and present an unacceptable backward slope between the two. You need only watch the personalities on TV chat shows fidgeting about in a vain attempt to get comfortable in these ultra-modern 'designer' chairs to understand the picture.

Our ancestors had much better ideas about furniture design. Try a reproduction Queen Anne wing armchair, a good Chesterfield or a Regency style dining chair and feel the difference. If all else fails, ask for a kitchen chair and at least you won't make your back pain worse.

Car seats are another area of violent controversy. There is only one factor to consider – are you comfortable in the driving seat? If not, don't fall for the advertising which describes adjustable lumbar supports, contoured seating, or any other jargon. If you are in pain, that seat is not for you. Before buying a car, try to borrow or hire a similar model for a few days first. Two miles up the road with an enthusiastic salesman beside you is hardly a fair test.

The doctor says he can't find anything wrong with my wife's back and he's given her valium to take. Is her pain all in the mind?

If your wife is in pain, then that pain is real. Sometimes the cause of back pain can be greatly aggravated by psychological factors. Mental stress, anxiety, fear and apprehension can all contribute to muscle tension. This in turn can give rise to back pain. If there is already an underlying back problem, then those psychosomatic factors will inevitably make matters worse.

The physical condition will create the mental problems which in turn can make the physical side even worse. A vicious circle ensues and to achieve a breakthrough in therapy it has to be broken somewhere. The short-term use of valium to help muscle relaxation can help but it is much more important to tackle the cause of the problem, not its effect. Massage, relaxation techniques, appropriate treatment and understanding will achieve far more than pills. The most potent remedy for your wife is TLC – Tender Loving Care. You must understand the difference between her type of psychosomatic (mind/body) problems which are absolutely real, and the fictitious pain of the true malingerer.

I've been told to give up sport in case I injure my back. It does hurt to play golf and tennis and, of course, sex is out of the question.

You must not give up your sporting activities. Not only are they very important for rehabilitating and strengthening your back, but regular exercise is vital to the proper care of your cardiovascular system (heart and circulation). Surprisingly, many top international athletes have back trouble, and they don't give up. The secret lies in correct maintenance of the muscles which support your spine. Also the way in which you use your back in sport is vital. You will understand more of that when you read the chapter on back fitness.

Not to have a normal healthy sex life is out of the question. Apart from the marital disasters that abstinence produces there are positive benefits, as well as pleasures, to be gained from normal sexual activity. During intercourse your body produces powerful chemicals which induce muscle relaxation and a wonderful sensation of peace and well-being in both partners. This deep relaxation helps relieve pain and discomfort in the affected area of your back. Furthermore, the movements of the pelvis provide gentle rhythmic exercise and so help restore better mobility to the spine.

Naturally, if your back hurts, you will not feel inclined to be a sexual gymnast. Whilst playing sport and being sexually active may produce some pain, this does not mean that you are likely to injure or damage your spine. The pain will certainly be muscular and caused by unaccustomed use, or faulty methods, producing stresses and strains that can be avoided.

The object of this book is to provide a practical guide for both partners which will show you how to enjoy sex in spite of back pain. In fact, the simple information and instructions will lead to an even fuller, more rewarding and satisfying sex life than before. Never doubt that there is sex after, and even during back pain. You can enjoy it yourself and you can certainly afford excitement, pleasure and satisfaction to your partner.

CHAPTER 2

Anatomy of the Spine and its Mechanics

Like your lawnmower or bicycle, you need to know a little about how your spine is put together in order to keep it in good order. With a car or lawnmower, you soon learn from the manual how often to change the oil, when to replace the spark plug, how to adjust the gears, how to remove a wheel, how to operate the machine properly, where all the parts are and what they are called, and above all, how to maintain the machine in good order, so as to provide a long and safe working life.

Secondly, bodies don't come with a guarantee and a workshop manual. Most people learn all about earthworms, cockroaches and dog fish at school, but virtually nothing about their own bodies. Before we move on to the Routine Service Guide for the Spine, we must first see how it is put together and how it works.

THE SPINE

The spine is a column of bones built one on top of the other like bricks and this column is divided into five distinct sections.

The overall shape of the spinal column is like a tall thin pyramid – smaller at the top, with the bones getting gradually larger, stronger and heavier at the bottom.

Spinal column

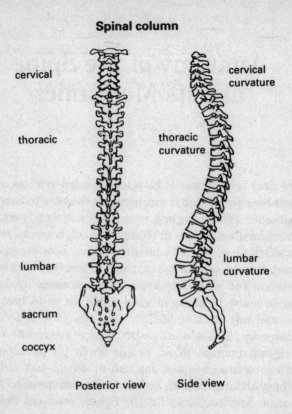

cervical

cervical curvature

thoracic

thoracic curvature

lumbar

lumbar curvature

sacrum

coccyx

Posterior view   Side view

Between each pair of bones, or vertebrae, is the infamous intervertebral disc which is mainly cartilage. The whole structure is supported by ligaments which act in much the same way as the guy ropes on a tent pole. The head, limbs and ribs are attached to the spine by more ligaments and muscles.

Each vertebra has a number of bony protuberances to which more muscles and ligaments are attached. These outcrops of bone join together at the back of the vertebra, forming the vertebral canal through which

16

the spinal cord passes, protected from injury by the arch of bone.

At the side of each pair of vertebrae is the foramen, a space through which the main spinal nerves and some smaller nerves can pass, issuing from the spinal cord, passing around the body and supplying all the bodily tissues.

NAMING OF PARTS

The neck or **cervical spine** is the top section which supports the head and consists of seven vertebrae. The chest or **thoracic spine** makes up the middle section of the back and consists of twelve bones to which are attached the twelve ribs on each side.

The lower back or **lumbar region** has the largest and strongest bones, since not only do they support the entire weight of the head, neck, arms and trunk, but these joints are also very flexible and must be able to withstand great stresses and strains. There are normally, but not always, five lumbar vertebrae.

The **sacrum**, a large triangular bone, forms the base upon which the spine is supported. This important bone is joined to the fifth lumbar vertebra at its top, and the huge bones of the pelvis at each side. These pelvic joints are the sacro-iliac joints, so often the cause of back pain. The sacrum is like the cornerstone in a brick archway, the downward pressure of the body weight pushes the wedge into its socket and maintains the rigid structure of the pelvis.

Attached to the tip of the sacrum is all that remains of the tail we once had. This tail, or **coccyx**, is only about one inch long and is made up of three or four segments. Injury to the coccyx can make sitting excruciating and even cause great pain during sexual intercourse.

Curvature of the spine

The normal curves of the back are essential to maintain fluid movement and even weight distribution. Any distortion of the normal shape of the spinal column can lead to excessive strain being placed on the muscle and ligament structures and this in turn produces pain.

Many patients are often terrified after being told they have a 'spinal curvature'. This conjures up dreadful images of progressive deformity leaving the patient a disabled cripple. This is hardly ever the case since most of these abnormal curves are mild and not progressive. Even the symptoms which they produce can be dealt with.

A few people are born with spinal abnormalities and some doctors believe that this is true of all cases of spinal curvature. Twenty years of experience have convinced me that this is absolutely untrue. Most of these abnormalities are acquired, either early on in life by children copying the posture of a parent (after all, we learn to walk, talk and eat by imitation) or they are occupational. Dentists, architects, potters and many musicians develop occupational curves in their spines.

The permanence of posture

The psychological part played in posture must never be overlooked. The way we stand and move is the externalisation of our own inner feelings and whether this is conscious or subconscious is irrelevant. To the experienced practitioner, this 'body language' provides useful clues. The dejected, depressed person will slump and stoop at the shoulders. He is 'carrying the weight of the world on his shoulders'.

The hyperactive, aggressive subject will be rigid, erect and move in a jerky and explosive manner. Both these psychological patterns will produce muscular and ligament stress that causes pain. The same is true of the tall child who stoops to be more like his friends; the short child

18

who stands extra tall and hyperextends his back; the over-developed young girl who rounds her shoulders to hide her breasts and even the young child subjected to repeated emotional stress who adopts the defensive attitude of bending forward at the hips with head forward. All these patterns eventually become the accepted posture and feel normal. They can all cause chronic back pain.

Curves

Lordosis, Kyphosis and **Scoliosis** are the three terms you will hear most often. These are the names of different curves.

Lordosis is the name given to the normal inward curve at the base of the spine and that in the neck region. These can be exaggerated, diminished, lost or reversed. **Kyphosis** is the normal outward curve of the thoracic spine, between the shoulders. The same abnormalities are possible. **Scoliosis** is a sideways curve which can occur at the cervical, thoracic or lumbar regions, and in fact is usually found in all three. This happens because in order to maintain the body's centre of gravity and the upright posture, your body will always try to keep your head directly over your tail. The cervical and lumbar regions of your back are the most mobile and hence those most commonly affected by back pain.

WHAT CAUSES BACK PAIN?

The human spine is built up of a series of functional components into a flexible articulated structure, and normal function of the whole depends entirely on the integrity of each part. The front part of the spine comprises the weight-bearing bony structure of the body of each vertebra, with a shock-absorbing disc between each pair of bones. The back portion contains the articulating facets, or joints, which control the directional movement of the spine, but do not carry any weight. The osteopath is directly concerned with the relationship between structure and function. By restoring normal structure he can ensure the return of normal function. This biodynamic relationship is the key to a strong healthy back.

To understand where and how back pain arises, we must consider the upright static posture and the complex movements of the spine in activity. Pain is always the result of irritation or inflammation of pain-sensitive tissues in the whole structure of the spine. Faulty posture or the wrong type of movement can cause irritation or inflammation and sometimes both and this leads to pain.

CHAPTER 3

The Quartet for Muscles, Ligaments, Joints and Nerves

There are four prime reasons for backache, and these can occur singly or in any combination:

1. A damaged or degenerated disc can bulge at the edges when under extreme pressure. This can squeeze against the posterior ligament of the spine which is pain-sensitive.
2. The rear portion of the vertebrae form the articular facets of the spinal joints. Like any other joint in the human body, the membrane which lines the inside of them is richly supplied with sensory nerves and can become swollen and inflamed. This results in pain.
3. Muscle spasm produced by faulty posture, injury or strain can itself cause pain. If there is also disc degeneration present, the vice-like pressure of the muscle spasm will cause disc compression and subsequent ligament pain as well.
4. Acute pain caused by pressure on a nerve root is also the fault of the degenerated disc. Usually in this type of back pain the wall of the disc loses its natural elastic quality and the soft jelly in the centre of the disc bulges out. A slight bulge or hernia presses on the posterior ligament as in type 1., but a more severe bulge, or a broken-off fragment of disc can cause pressure on the

nerve tissue and acute pain. This pain sometimes travels down one leg, or both, giving rise to the condition known as sciatica. This can result in numbness, pins and needles, abnormal nerve reflexes and loss of muscle strength. This type of nerve pain often produces pain in the other areas as well – ligaments, joints, and muscles.

TREATMENT FOR BACK PAIN

It is safe to say that normal posture and normal activity in a normal spine are most unlikely to produce pain. But abnormal posture or movement can cause pain in an otherwise normal spine and are almost certain to do so in an abnormal one. In order to relieve back pain, and much more importantly, to prevent its regular occurrence, the course of treatment and preventative measures need to be based on an exact knowledge of the patient's condition.

The practitioner must know the where, when and how of the pain. For this reason the osteopathic case history must be exhaustive. Examination of the patient sitting, standing, walking, lying and being moved passively are essential ingredients. Even the patient's shoes must be looked at closely as they give a truly objective picture of the patient's weight distribution when walking. If it is possible to reproduce the patient's pain by a particular position or movement, then the osteopath will understand the way in which that pain is produced in the patient.

It's very common for patients to want a specific diagnosis of the exact cause of their back pain. But sadly this is often not possible. To be honest, I believe that in some ways it's preferable to avoid attaching precise labels as these are often arrived at by a process of elimination and guesswork and once written it's as though they were engraved on tablets of stone on the patient's medical

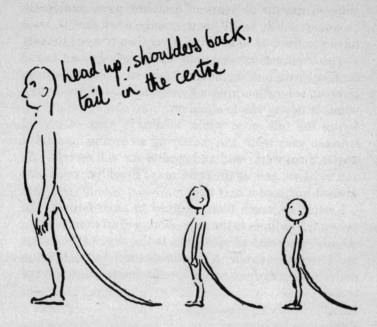

head up, shoulders back, tail in the centre

record. If the diagnosis was incorrect, then that patient will struggle from practitioner to practitioner, from hospital to hospital, from therapist to therapist, all of whom are likely to accept the specific diagnosis. Their forms of treatment may vary but they are probably all going to be treating the same condition, and it may be the wrong condition.

Naturally patients have been conditioned to believe that medicine is an exact science and, consequently, they need an exact diagnosis. Low back pain, lumbago, sciatica or wear and tear are probably not acceptable. If the sufferer did but know it, they are probably better off with these rather vague and old-fashioned descriptions as they are more likely to be looked at with a fresh eye by different practitioners. Be wary of the expert who, within five minutes of seeing you for the first time after you've suffered months or years of disabling pain, confidently pronounces: 'Oh yes, I know exactly what that is, we'll have you fixed up in no time.' They then proceed to twist you up like a reef knot on their manipulating couch, hover over you with a swinging pendulum on a piece of string, creep up behind you with a hypodermic full of who knows what, or advise you to stand on your head in the garden facing the full moon whilst holding a piece of crystal between your teeth and muttering an arcane mantra! If any of them work, well and good. Some will certainly do you no harm, and, as the residents of Brooklyn would say: 'It can't hurt and it may help.'

I would be much more inclined to have faith in the person who admits to the impossibility of an exact diagnosis, who expresses an opinion as to the most likely causes and is prepared to offer a holistic approach to treating the entire person rather than a specific magic bullet form of therapy.

Backs can be bizarre

Most patients and many doctors fail to understand that problems arising from the structure of the spine may manifest themselves as symptoms in distant parts of the body. Pain may often be referred to other regions – sciatica or pain in the leg as a result of lesions in the lower part of the spine or brachial neuritis, pain in the arm caused by problems in the neck or shoulder. These two are common and well recognised, but what are not so well recognised are some of the other conditions related to back pain or some of the more bizarre symptoms, often mimicking internal problems, which can also be the result of spinal dysfunction.

Tennis elbow, pain in the hand and fingers, shoulder pain, giddiness, tinnitus, throat and voice problems, pain in the ear, and recurrent headaches can all be linked to problems in the neck. Most osteopaths see countless

24

patients who have been treated for all these conditions but never had their neck properly examined, let alone X-rayed. Don't be fobbed off with yet another bottle of pills, but suggest tactfully to your GP that it might not be a bad idea to see if there's anything wrong with the neck as the last three different prescriptions didn't seem to help at all.

MRS M's STORY

If you think this sounds like an exaggeration, then let me tell you about Mrs. M. She happens to be my aunt and a few years ago collapsed in the middle of her local High Street, was rushed to hospital and diagnosed as having suffered a severe heart attack. I had been treating auntie for several years as she suffered from severe arthritis in her neck. She'd been a serious gymnast in her youth, a sport which predisposes to spinal joint problems in later life. Although in her late sixties she was still an extremely fit and active woman, having kept up her exercise by swimming at least three times a week and walking every day. She'd never shown any sign of heart disease, and I knew that she followed a healthy diet and neither smoked nor drank alcohol.

The family were summoned to her bedside at the intensive care unit of a major London teaching hospital, and we were warned to expect the worst. I had a quiet word with the doctor on duty and asked if anybody had looked at her neck or indeed if any proper investigations had yet been done to discover the extent of her heart attack. His answer was no and no. She'd only been in the hospital for three hours and although she had regained consciousness, they now had her on a drip and she was wired up to a battery of machines. They were awaiting results of the tests. I could have told him the answer. Twenty-four hours later she was back home wearing a neck collar, all the heart tests having proved negative. In older people with arthritis of the neck, twisting the head can obstruct the artery that supplies the brain, and cause a sudden severe fainting episode. It's surprisingly common and surprisingly often mistaken for a heart attack.

Injury, arthritis or disc problems in the middle part of the back – the thoracic spine – are a very frequent cause of pain radiating round the side of the chest wall between the ribs and behind the breast bone. The same pain can be caused by abnormalities at the joint where the rib joins on to the side of the vertebra. In both these situations the resulting chest pain can easily lead to the suspicion of heart disease, blood tests, ECGs and all the stress caused by this type of investigation.

WHICH WAY TO TURN?

Many difficulties arise due to the over-specialisation of medicine. It may sound like a joke to say that a specialist is someone who knows more and more about less and less, but I'm sure the day is not far off when you might see one doctor for the left ear and another for the right. No, that's only a joke, but it's not so far from the truth. Women have particular problems in this area, as the successful outcome of treatment depends entirely on which speciality their GP chooses to refer them to. Pain in the lower abdomen may be caused by problems with the womb or ovaries, and similarly, pain in the back may be caused in the same way. Back problems, on the other hand, may also lead to pain in the abdomen. If the first specialist happens to be a gynaecologist and the problem starts in the back, the poor patient is on a hiding to nothing. On the other hand, if the GP's first choice is an orthopaedic surgeon for the back pain and it's caused by a misplaced uterus, the patient might well endure six months of fruitless physiotherapy and endless anti-inflammatory drugs before she finally sees a gynaecologist. Yet another desperate plea for a holistic look at the entire patient, not just the bits.

Many patients with stomach pain can be subjected to the most unpleasant investigations which reveal nothing. It's only then that somebody thinks to look at the lower spine which is frequently the cause of referred pain to the abdomen. In this situation a meticulous case history would reveal that the pain is never related to eating or not eating, to particular foods, to an excess of coffee, tea, alcohol, or Mars bars. In fact, it has no relation to the patient's digestive function whatsoever. Q.E.D. it's unlikely to be anything to do with a digestive problem.

Tricks of the trade

If you bear the cross of back pain here is some general advice which you should follow as a matter of course. Some of these topics are covered in much greater detail elsewhere in the book, but as a starting point these are the key factors which you must be aware of.

1. Keep your weight down, be ever vigilant about bending, lifting, stretching and twisting as these are the movements which put your back at the greatest risk. The worst of all is a combination of twisting and bending or stretching which places enormous shearing stresses on the spine. Use your thigh and lower leg muscles, not the back muscles, for lifting. Avoid heavy loads and when carrying keep the load as close to your body as possible – a baby lifted over the top of the cot with straight arms exerts five times its weight on the base of your spine.

2. No matter what your age a programme of regular back exercises will help to maintain the support of strong muscles and the mobility of your spinal joints. Any osteopath or chiropractor will show you the correct exercises to do, and there is a complete set of them for both treatment and prevention in Chapters 6 and 7.

3. Any seat that you occupy for long periods of time must be a vital factor in both the cause and the relief of backache. The soft, non-supportive, very low armchair that you fall asleep in in front of the TV screen every night; the office chair which glues you to the VDU for six hours a day, or the car seat which offers no lumbar or side support and puts you behind steering wheels and pedals which are offset to the side – all need close scrutiny.

The armchair should have a high straight back and a firm seat, the office chair must be adjustable for height, rake and back support, and you should have a footstool for complete comfort. Choose your car for the seat, rather than its colour or performance. Price is seldom a factor in relation to good driving seats. I've tried some of the most expensive vehicles on the road and been appalled by the quality of their seats. Many years ago I bought an old fourth-hand Toyota Supra as it had the best seat I'd ever found in a standard production car. I'm now driving my fifth of the same model, just because of the seats.

Employers have a legal duty to provide work stations which put you at the least risk of postural problems, eye strain, headaches, stiff necks, pains in the shoulders and arms, repetitive strain injuries and backache. These can all be avoided by putting together work surfaces and seats of the right sort and your local osteopath or chiropractor will be able to advise you as to the best posture for your particular work.

HOW TO FIND AN OSTEOPATH OR CHIROPRACTOR

If backache strikes, don't just go to bed and lie there, the latest research shows that two weeks of bed rest can actually make matters worse not better. Ask your GP to recommend a local osteopath or chiropractor as he is most likely to know the best practitioners in your area, or look in the Yellow Pages and make sure you choose a practitioner who is properly trained and qualified. There are lots of frighteningly bad weekend courses which turn out practitioners with little or no clinical experience and questionable diagnostic skills. They represent a real threat as their lack of general medical education and inability to arrive at a diagnosis may lead to delays in seeking specialist medical attention for serious underlying problems.

There are a number of schools which run adequate courses but my personal preference is for those practitioners trained at one of the schools recognised by the General Council and Register of Osteopaths and whose graduates are entitled to use the style 'Member of the Register of Osteopaths (MRO)'. The same is true for chiropractors and again I would only feel happy recommending a graduate of the Anglo-European College of Chiropractic or one of its associated establishments which entitle graduates to use the letters 'MBCA' (Member of the British Chiropractic Association).

WHEN THE PAIN STRIKES

There are things you can do to help even when acute back pain strikes. Forty-eight hours in bed, either flat on your back with a pillow under your knees, or on your side with a pillow between your knees and drawn up into the foetal position, are the only postures which you should adopt. The more complete your bedrest the more likely you are to recover quickly, especially if the pain is caused by disc pressure. When you are not weight-bearing the intervertebral discs absorb fluid and swell. This helps to separate the vertebrae and relieve nerve root pressure. Men should pee into a bottle but trying to use a bedpan if you are a woman or if you need to have your bowels open is likely to cause more spinal stress than struggling to the lavatory. Make sure someone is there to help you.

The application of alternate hot and cold packs will stimulate the circulation and encourage healing. Use a hot water bottle wrapped in a towel and a large bag of frozen peas wrapped in a thin tea cloth and apply them alternately for two minutes at a time for at least twenty minutes, two or three times a day. Again, it's much better if someone else is there to do this for you. Always finish with the frozen peas. They make an ideal ice-pack as once you've given the bag a good shake they can be moulded exactly to fit the area required, but do mark the bag with a large red cross so that no one eats them. They're going to be in and out of the freezer for several days.

Once the acute phase has worn off then you can start to be a little more active, alternating between lying down and pottering about. Do not stand and do not sit in your soft armchair but walk around or sit for short periods in an upright kitchen chair. Any of the heat-generating rubs like Tiger Balm or Ralgex may help and don't be afraid to use your normal pain-killers, taking care not to exceed the recommended dose.

Don't consume large amounts of alcohol or smoke. Surprisingly, smoking adversely affects the circulation to the spinal structures by constricting the tiny blood vessels which supply them, and consequently delaying proper healing of local tissue damage. A small amount of alcohol is quite a good muscle relaxant but large quantities also have an adverse effect on the circulation and cause dehydration which will not help a damaged disc.

Once you start to feel even more comfortable, gentle traction can speed up the healing process even more. You can apply this to your own back very simply by hanging from a bar placed inside a door frame – most sports shops sell these, or you can reach up and behind you to hold onto the banister supports of a staircase and just lift your feet off the ground using your arm muscles.

The first exercise you should take is getting your body into a warm swimming pool. It doesn't matter if you can't swim, just moving gently in the water and getting your spinal muscles to stretch and relax is enough to help your back on its way to recovery.

If by the third day you are still in acute pain, you must get professional help, either from your GP or osteopath. If you've had the problem before, it's likely that you already know a local practitioner in which case get help as soon as possible.

CHAPTER 4

The Battle Against
Back Pain

THE PAIN

This begins when a normal healthy person of any age and either sex develops back pain. It makes no difference which type of pain or what area of the spine is involved. Psychosomatic pain doesn't make the struggle any easier. It does not matter if you are 67 and have arthritis, or 24 and hurt your back climbing mountains in the Andes. If your back hurts then you are locked into a lifelong struggle with your back as the battle ground.

It's not much different from the ancient Roman games with you cast in the role of the gladiator. Whether it's thumbs up or thumbs down depends on you, with, of course, a little help from your osteopath. You may win or lose and most sufferers tend to waver from one side to the other until they learn how to live in harmony with their back – how to do everything possible to protect it and nothing that will aggravate it.

In the early days the struggle is at its most difficult as your first encounter strikes like a thunderbolt from the blue leaving you with acute and disabling pain. In an instant you are transformed from a normal active and busy person to a helpless, dependent bedridden patient who can't even get your own socks on, let alone stand up long enough to go to the toilet. Visions of a wheelchair

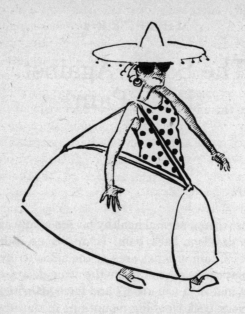

float before your eyes, and a life of permanent invalidity stretches out before you.

If you're lucky this state of panic and depression soon passes. A few days bedrest, strong pain-killers, and most first time acute sufferers are on the mend. A few tentative steps around the garden. A short walk to the shops or the 'local' and then back to work.

At this point you face the first major decision. Do you go back to life as normal, give up all the things you enjoy in a fit of terror, or do you seek more help?

The stoics amongst you will just carry on as normal but in the long term this can prove disastrous. The second group are in for a rocky ride from the start and the outlook for them is decidedly bleak but it is the third group who will get the thumbs up at the end of the day.

Why are the groups so different? The stoics in the first group forge ahead and make good progress, until – yes you guessed – another thunderbolt. This time a bit worse, it takes longer to get better and they are more frightened second time around. They then lapse into the type two attitude and give up everything. But all is not lost. They can still join the third group and learn how to overcome their back problem. The trick is your psychological approach to this intellectual stage of back pain.

Group two have the greatest problems, since they have been treated very unfairly in the early stages of their condition. What they need if they're going to stand any chance of getting better is the best advice they can find. If you're in this group, beware, you've become a negative time-server just waiting for the inevitable. If you were sitting in my treatment room you'd be saying, 'The doctor says I've got to learn to live with it' or 'The physiotherapist says "what can you expect at your age?" ' or 'The surgeon says nothing can be done'. What the surgeon actually means is that your back is not bad enough for surgery, but doesn't take the time to explain.

Phrases like these are all part of the medical profession's Fifth Column activities. They undermine your confidence, take away whatever positive thoughts you've still got left about your physical condition and leave you with every chance of being a permanent martyr to backache.

If you're in group three then you're off to a flying start. You'll get professional help right from the outset and you'll learn the right techniques which will enable you to start out on the road to recovery and victory. Any chance of success depends on knowing the right techniques, but in order to maximise your chances of returning to a full normal and active life you must know the rules and above all you need the correct psychological approach so that you are neither over-confident nor excessively timid in your attitude to physical activity.

In Billy Jean King's first serious tennis lesson the coach said to her, 'Winning isn't everything – it's the only thing.'

And she has won more Wimbledon titles than any other player. You must want to win your battle against back pain above all else. You must psyche yourself up into believing that you can and will win.

If you stay with me to the end of this book I'll teach you all the Rules you need to know so that you can get yourself back to strength. Once you know them, and you are prepared to practise regularly, exercise every day and develop the right positive attitudes, you will win back, feet and hands down.

MAIN OBJECTIVES

1. To relieve pain.
2. To restore movement and activity.
3. To minimise the chances of repeated attacks.
4. To reduce the level of any residual loss of function.
5. To prevent the condition becoming chronic.
6. To return to a normal social, sporting and working life.
7. To encourage the resumption of your normal physical relationship which is not only beneficial but nice as well as naughty!

RULES

Winning is the only thing
You must cultivate the right, positive mental attitude. You must be determined to win.

Make time – 12 minutes a day is all you need
You need a high level of skill to build back strength and this type of expertise does not come naturally. You must work for it, and that means practice, practice and more practice. You would not expect to be an expert golfer just

because you bought an expensive set of clubs. Give up 12 minutes a day for your exercises and your back will give you years of uncomplaining service.

Know when – and when not
The idea that attack is the best form of defence is not always true when dealing with back pain. There are pains which you have to work through with your exercises and there are pains which are a warning to stop everything. If you don't know when to go on to the defensive and protect your back you'll suffer just as much as if you never attack your problem at its roots. Always remember that the best strategy for an acute attack of back pain is REST.

One Christmas morning I was called to the home of a well-known TV personality. 'Come at once,' said his panic-stricken wife, 'he's on the bathroom floor and I can't move him.' Sure enough, there he was, head between the loo and the wash basin, feet by the bath, in acute pain and terrified.

'Thank God you're here,' he said, 'you must do something quickly, my show starts on TV again in two days.'

We got him back to bed. I showed him exactly how to lie so as to give the maximum relaxation to his poor back and warned him not to get up for anything, not even to go to the bathroom.

'But aren't you going to *do* anything?' he said desperately.

'I've done it,' I replied. 'You see, only Nature heals, the practitioner just helps the process along, and if you want to do your next show, follow my instructions and I'll be back tomorrow.'

Sure enough he was much better twenty-four hours later and no one seeing his programme the next day would have been any the wiser.

To master the 'when and when not' rule you need to understand when to rest your back, when to be mobile and when to really work the joints and muscles of your spine. Failure to grasp this rule fully can result in repeated acute and painful episodes or a life of boring, unfulfilling chronic inactivity. Either way, you're the loser and martyrdom looms onto the horizon.

Know exactly what your problem is
How you tackle your back pain depends on a proper diagnosis.

You will have to make some drastic changes in the way you use your back and these vary with the cause. What is essential for inflamed joints will not always be right for a degenerated disc or muscle strain.

If no one has told you *exactly* what is wrong with your back, then ask. It is, after all, your body, your back and your pain, and no practitioner should advise a course of treatment without arriving at a diagnosis, even if it is one of the exclusion of serious underlying problems. If he knows, so should you. If he doesn't, then he should be finding out, but sometimes back pain can be an insidious and mystifying condition. It can be disguised by other symptoms, pain in other parts of the body and a confusing and unpredictable course. For all these reasons an exact diagnosis with a specific label is not always possible.

I fully understand that your defences may be down, you are after all in pain, probably frightened, certainly nervous, but you will only get better if you start NOW with:

Responsibility
The patient who gets back to strength quickest recognises very early on that it is no good just putting yourself in the hands of others. Most modern medicine assumes total control of, and responsibility for, the patient. *You must not allow this to happen.* The penalty for abdicating all responsibility to any practitioner is almost guaranteed failure. If you take no responsibility for yourself the

chances are that you'll turn into one of the host of back sufferers who become dependent on their therapist, the drugs, the treatment, even the seductive comforts of their regular visit to the surgery. If you let this happen to you, you'll never have an incentive to help yourself.

Successful therapy needs a balanced working relationship between patient and practitioner. The therapist must insist that the patient accepts responsibility for his own care and rehabilitation. Many approaches to back pain can, and do, produce rapid alleviation of the symptoms. Only continuous vigilance and hard work by the patient pay the long-term dividends which guarantee the best odds in favour of recovery.

Survive against the odds

The odds against you are tremendous and no self-respecting gambler would ever bet on you. The secret of success is that you must bet on yourself – and no hedging with each way bets either. Have faith in your own strength of character, bet on yourself to win and you will overcome the odds and succeed.

Eighty per cent of all people will suffer some period of back pain, and after your first episode of acute back trouble you are 50 per cent more likely to get a second attack than you were to get the first. You can learn to shorten the odds in your favour, but you must be aware of unforced errors which will always count against you. You can realise every punter's greatest dream and be the winning outsider. But if you're going to beat the backache bookie you have got to make changes to your own personal:

Life-style

One of the most significant rules that you must follow is the life-style challenge. It's no good refusing to make changes and carrying on as if nothing had happened. It's also no good giving up everything – work, hobbies, sport, and always sex (see Chapter 5). Both these life-styles are negative and counter-productive.

The correct life-style changes involve learning to live with your back. You've got it for life and there are no factory exchange units available. Winners form a symbiotic relationship with their spines, that is, they live together to their mutual advantage. You will learn how to lift and carry; how to make the bed and clean the bath; how to sit, stand or use machines at work; how to drive your car; what to do at the first signs of trouble; how to minimise all the risks you encounter during daily life; how to live a rich and full social and domestic life, and above all how to care for your own particular back problem. These changes will put you firmly on the road to victory and enable you to get the most out of life.

Work, Sports and Hobbies
There are very few occupations to which the back sufferer should not return. By building up all the supportive structures of the spine, improving its flexibility and learning how to use it correctly, most patients can return to their normal job with very few problems. The same is true of nearly all sports and hobbies, but do use your common sense.

I am certain that I could judge the seasons of the year, even if I never set foot outside my consulting room, just by the back problems that patients bring to me. The first fine weekend after Christmas brings the gardeners; the first fine days of spring produce the DIY brigade who can't resist getting out the ladders; next come the casual tennis players who have not hit a ball for six months and play for three hours the first time out. They are followed by the pre-summer holiday brigade who dash off to aerobics classes after trying on last year's swimsuits; autumn brings the leaf sweepers and the 'One last mow before winter' brigade; followed by the 'I haven't been on skis since leaving school' contingent, and finally, the harassed mums who get no help at all lifting a huge turkey with stuffing, potatoes and a red hot dish out of a badly designed oven fixed in quite the wrong position for her.

You can do almost anything you enjoy but to get back to strength you must be properly prepared. If you have not been in the garden for three or four months, you would expect your back to ache after three hours of digging in heavy, wet soil. If you have never had a 'bad back' you will take a hot bath, moan and groan for a few days and ignore the discomfort. The back patient panics and fears that irreparable harm has been done. This is most unlikely, but like the frog trying to climb up the inside of the well you will slide back a bit and delay your recovery. These problems can be avoided with care. Remember *hurt* is not the same as *harm*. Many activities may hurt a bit, but done correctly will cause no harm to your back.

Mind or Body

This rule states that unless you are a true malingerer (a very rare, almost extinct species) it does not matter a damn whether your pain originates in mind or body. It is still your pain and moreover it is a brave, or foolhardy, practitioner who tries drawing rigid dividing lines.

What does matter, if you are going to beat this problem, is that you ask yourself some honest questions about your back. You need to understand the psychological part of your problem, and there nearly always is one. That's the only way you can fight to overcome it and get back to strength.

Broadly speaking, there are two psychological responses to back pain, either Martyrdom or Total Collapse. The question is why.

The **martyr** is often the self-employed professional or the high-powered executive who feels that his or her total enterprise will crumble like a house of cards if they are absent for more than a few hours. The same is often true of 'Good old Mum'. She has always struggled through every crisis. She doesn't go to bed when she gets colds or flu, and after all there's the washing to do, John's rugby kit, Jenny's new outfit to alter for the party and Dad is bringing some friends over for a drink and sandwiches. So how can she possibly go to bed for two or three days?

The **collapsers** find themselves the centre of attention and care, sometimes for the only time in their lives. Consequently they grow more and more reluctant to relinquish the pain which produces this strange, but pleasant, response from their spouse, family or work colleagues. The martyr must realise the long term dangers of soldiering on; the collapser the futility of prolonged invalidity. But martyrs sometimes collapse!

Both patient and practitioner are faced with a 'chicken and egg' problem. Have the psychological pressures on the patient led to the condition which now relieves them of some onerous burdens? It is true that life can send you what you need. If you really need to get away from it all and turn your back on a difficult situation, life will often take matters in hand – though not always in the manner you would choose. Or has the pain and disability of the problem resulted in a personality change, which in turn makes physical matters worse?

Sexual activity is one sphere where those questions are of the utmost importance. In an unsatisfactory relationship, especially where one partner wishes to punish the other, withholding sexual favours is a potent weapon. Having an apparently good reason to refuse sexual advances makes it so much easier to say 'Not tonight darling, my back is killing me.' If you do not want to have sexual intercourse with your partner and are unable to resolve the problem in your relationship, then you have a deep-rooted interest in perpetuating your back problem.

There is no sound medical reason for abstaining from sex *just* because you have a back problem. If there are other reasons which you cannot or will not talk over with your partner, then that's your problem. But you had better do something about it now, because if you are reading this book, it won't be long before your other half does. Then you are going to have some quick explaining to do!

CHAPTER 5

Sex Rules, OK!

During thirty-five years of dealing with other people's back problems, as well as my own, I have NEVER told a patient to stop sexual activities. Apart from the first forty-eight hours of an acute disc rupture, there is not one situation in which sex would make your back worse. If you are able to overcome the practical problems and modify your approach to intercourse, you will certainly be a winner in the Back Game. There aren't many physical games where men and women play together on an equal footing, where strength doesn't really count, where the ideal result is a draw and where a third party – the Back Brat – could sabotage either of the players, if not both. It doesn't matter if you are Torvill and Dean, Daley Thompson and Fatima Whitbread, André Agassi and Monica Seles or the best pair of couch potatoes in the world, this is the most important game you will ever play. Before we get to specific instructions you must grasp the principles involved.

Let's assume that you *want* to make love to your partner and it's your back which hurts. After two or three tries which cause excruciating pain, you give up, and decide that the possible ecstasy is just not worth the very real agony. At first your partner is concerned, understanding and sympathetic. This does not last. It won't be long before the resentment and frustrations begin to show and unless you can do something positive to remedy the situation, there is a rocky path ahead. Of course, sex is not everything in any relationship, but it is a fundamental need in human beings and an expression of love, affection, respect and care for your partner. It's also a supreme way of washing away the petty squabbles and trials and tribulations of everyday life which we all endure.

If it is your partner who is suffering from the Back Brat and you are aggravating their pain, then your advances will soon be rebuffed and it's you who will start resenting the situation.

'Is it really his back or do you think he doesn't want me any more? Perhaps he's got a girlfriend that I don't know about?'

This is such a sad, but frequent question that is asked in my office all too often. In some cases the backache really is no more than an excuse, but nearly always the reason is just plain ignorance. If your sex life is confined to alternate Saturdays (if there's no football on the telly and the lads aren't coming round for a few jars and a game of cards), then it is not surprising that you have not been able to discuss your difficulties together.

Do not despair, help is at hand, because once you have mastered the intricacies of The Game and have got through the heats to the Final, a whole new world awaits you. No more furtive, embarrassed and usually painful sex for you. Some frank, open, plain talking about, and not around, your difficulties will give you a new perspective on the joys of sex. As a human being you are entitled to expect a normal healthy and active sex life. As a back sufferer, you NEED one. Firstly, because to give up sex is an admission of failure and the first step on the slippery slope to chronic illness, defeatism and a loss of your own sense of self-esteem. These all create the kind of psychological pressures which cause tension, stress and inevitably make your condition worse.

Secondly, during intercourse your body produces chemical substances known as endorphins. These occur in the brain and are your own in-built pain-killers. The release of endorphins relieves pain and enables you to achieve more spinal and muscular mobility. This increase in activity has a positive and beneficial effect on all back problems, whether in the neck, middle or lower components of your spine, and this improvement in your freedom of movement, coupled with the relaxing 'afterglow' of sexual activity, promotes your body's own healing process. It is a fact that if you suffer from any back complaint Sex is Good, but More Sex is Better.

Before warming up for the Game you must come to a good mutual understanding with your partner. This is not the situation that calls for swinging on the chandelier, jumping off wardrobes or any other sexual gymnastics. In the early stages you need to establish a healthy lead over your opponent, so take it nice and gently. Explore each other's strengths and weaknesses, but don't be too adventurous. There will be a lifetime to experiment once you have overcome all the dirty tricks of the Back Brat, and he's got plenty of those up his sleeve.

Make absolutely certain that you and your partner know just what you can and can't manage without real discomfort. Help each other by being aware of the problems, being gentle, caring and patient. Nothing is more of a sexual turn-off for man or woman than severe pain at the wrong moment. Some players enjoy a certain degree of pain in later stages of the game, but not the sort that comes from a damaged disc pressing on a nerve root. Bear in mind that your body's endorphins will relieve your own pain as sexual excitement mounts, but don't get too carried away and over-adventurous as you may regret it the next morning.

Never forget that hurt does not mean harm. You may suffer the odd twinge and discomfort during your exploratory moves around the pitch, but as long as you are not going to fall off the kitchen table, garden swing, or down the stairs you are unlikely to cause any damage to your back or your partner's.

As with all sports, the best players are fit, and you must get your back and body fit for the game by training as seriously as any Olympic athlete. Before any serious sexual activity you should start the exercise programme in Chapter 6. As you develop your back support and abdominal muscles you will find that you can be more vigorous and adventurous without pain or difficulty. Practice makes perfect, so don't get stuck into the same old routines. Experiment and initiative are the keys to victory and with plenty of patience and practice you will be a star player, have a great time together and beat the Back Brat into three pinfalls or a submission.

Forewarned is forearmed, so follow the simple detailed rules which you will have to study, understand and remember if you are going to win the Game and vanquish the Back Brat

BACK TO BED

Bed is not the only place to play this game, but with your problem, some care and common sense in the choice of playing field are mandatory. The home team normally has the advantage in all games, so until you are a real expert it is probably safer to play on familiar territory.

The bed should not be too small, you don't want to fall out onto your already painful back; nor should it be too soft since this will not provide adequate spinal support. Layers of heavy blankets and tightly tucked in 'hospital' sheets will limit your freedom of movement. The height of the bed is not crucial, though climbing up to a Victorian brass splendour, or down to a Japanese futon might cause problems. Make sure you have a few spare pillows since some extra support can make all the difference.

Get your clothes off first, if you can, otherwise ask for help. Do not be vain about this. Your partner would much rather give you a hand to remove your shoes, socks, tights or skin-hugging jeans than spend yet another night nursing your muscle spasm. It is also very awkward trying to get your Y-fronts off under the bedclothes if you are not fairly mobile.

ON THE WHAT?

All players in this game have their favourite venues, but here are a few suggestions as to where and when not to play. Most modern furniture is not ideal as it tends to be too soft and unstable. If you've got a firm sofa which is long enough and wide enough, it can be used to good effect – 18th-century cabinet-makers had wonderful designs for fornicating couches and I've seen one that used to reside in a royal palace! A high-backed, wooden rocking chair is excellent for some players as the back support is good and the rocking motion reduces the amount of muscular effort needed. A strong, softly upholstered stool, such as you would use for a dressing-table, can also be a useful piece of furniture, as can a straight-backed, well-made and upholstered chair without arms.

There is nothing wrong with the floor either, but make sure you have a good thick carpet or two or three blankets to lie on. The room should be warm and draught-free as nothing will stiffen up your back muscles as quickly as an icy north wind blowing under the door. It's worth bearing in mind that whilst the romantic notion of soft candlelight and a bearskin rug in front of the log fire is beautiful, reality may strike when you try to get up, and put rather a large dent in your 'last of the great lovers' image.

Cars are another ball game altogether. It's one thing

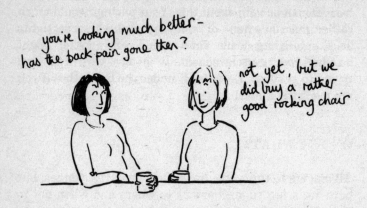

if you have a Rolls Royce or a Cadillac, quite another if your pride and joy is a Mini. Don't forget the true story of the couple in an MG Midget. His back went into spasm at the crucial moment. The fire brigade were summoned by a passing Good Samaritan and the only way to get the poor man out was by cutting the top off the car. The unfortunate lady was left with the task of explaining to her husband just what had happened to her brand new car!

If you are new to the game it's probably safer only to play at home to begin with and broaden your horizons as you become more accomplished and confident.

TAKING UP YOUR POSITION ON THE COURT

The following examples are based on the general principles of back care. They are *not* rigid instructions. You may find some of them good for you and others not. If you find any particular position too painful, don't carry on regardless just because the book says it's OK. Your back is unique to you and you may find positions of your own which are more suitable, or you may also find ways of adopting the ones described that suit you better.

You must always bear in mind that it is not only your back which must be considered as no matter which partner has been attacked by the Back Brat, simply finding a position which does not cause pain is not enough. You only win at this game if you achieve comfortable AND enjoyable sex. And that means enjoyable for both participants.

OVERWEIGHT?

A large stomach gets in the way during lovemaking, and makes some of the most suitable positions for the back game much more difficult to achieve. If the thin partner is the back sufferer, supporting an 18-stone lover is not really conducive to comfort.

A one-week, healthy eating plan will be found at the end of this chapter (see p52). Follow it and if you're seriously overweight you will see the pounds drop off. Stick to it for a month and you could lose the best part of a stone, which will not only help in this fun part of the Back Game, but will dramatically increase your chances of long-term victory over the Back Brat. Every extra pound you carry creates more pressure on your spine. Just imagine that extra stone as 28 half-pound packs of lard piled up on your dressing-table – in fact, it's not a bad idea to put them there and throw them away as the weight goes down. If you had all those packs in a shopping bag which you carried around with you all day, how would you feel by the time you got home? Just because it's spread all over your body doesn't reduce the toll that extra weight takes in terms of fatigue, joint strain and increased back pain.

Obesity is not good for lovers or back sufferers. If you

are overweight, you lose out on both counts, so do something about it now. Seriously fat men and women have statistically more back problems than their slimmer counterparts. Very overweight people with back pain tend to get even fatter – the pain prevents exercise and encourages them to be even more sedentary. However, I've no intention of encouraging anyone to become an obsessive slimmer. Being underweight leads to a shorter life expectancy than being moderately overweight. We're talking here about people who are more than 15–20 per cent above their ideal weight. It's particularly dangerous for women to be underweight as it interferes with their menstrual cycle, can be a cause of infertility and without doubt increases the risk of osteoporosis (brittle bone disease) and fractures in later life. It's worth remembering that over 50 per cent of women who fracture a hip in their seventies never lead an independent life again. Think about that before you try the next lunatic and unhealthy diet drink, meal replacement or 800 calorie a day diet plan.

HEALTHY EATING PLAN FOR THE SERIOUSLY OVERWEIGHT

We are all constantly bombarded from all sides with endless advice on how to lose weight, stay slim and be healthy. Every newspaper, woman's magazine and countless radio and TV programmes urge everyone to think thin. We are all targets for the multi-million pound slimming business which is more concerned with extracting pounds from pockets than it is with the nation's health. Unless you are grossly obese you are almost certainly better off staying as you are than making your life a misery by trying to reach the mythical 'ideal weight'. But if you have been attacked by the Back Brat and you are considerably overweight, then losing some of those extra pounds is a vital step on the road to victory.

Most of the dietary advice you see will include worthless pills, unhealthy meal substitutes or extreme diets based on pseudoscience and hocus pocus. If you have gained an extra inch or two because the Back Brat has made you less active than normal, and this makes you feel uncomfortable and not able to wear your favourite clothes, then here's a simple, healthy one-week eating plan that provides good nutrition, happy eating and real food. It's a way of eating that will compensate for too much time spent resting and too much 'comfort stuffing' of too many sweets and chocolates, too many cakes and biscuits and too many spoons of sugar in the tea. You won't be hungry, you will be healthy and you will lose pounds if you need to.

MONDAY

Breakfast
Baked beans on toast with a grilled tomato; a cup of tea or coffee with semi-skimmed milk. Have either drink with breakfast every day.

Light meal
A large portion of coleslaw made with red, white and green cabbage, carrots, sultanas, onion, apple, plain yogurt, a little olive oil and a tablespoon of cider vinegar, with a small cup of cottage cheese and a piece of fresh fruit.

Main meal
Chicken breast (skin removed) covered with a sliced courgette, thin strips of red pepper, a little garlic, the juice

of a lemon, half a glass of dry white wine and quarter of a pint of vegetable stock (from a cube) cooked in a covered casserole for 30 minutes at 175°C/350°F/gas mark 4, with carrots and parsnips mashed together. A baked apple (cooked in the oven at the same time). Remote the core, cut off the bottom quarter, put it back in the hole and stuff with 1 oz ground almonds mixed with orange juice, sprinkled with a little cinnamon and nutmeg.

TUESDAY

Breakfast
Porridge with half water, half skimmed milk, a slice of wholemeal toast with a little butter and honey.

Light meal
A large bowl of vegetable, bean and barley soup – 1 oz pot barley, 1½ pints water, 4 sliced carrots, 1 chopped turnip, 2 sliced leeks, 2 sticks celery, 1 chopped onion, 1 tsp tomato purée, black pepper, bring them to the boil and simmer for 45 minutes. Add a can of kidney, butter, haricot or any other sort of beans, cook for another 5 minutes to make six large portions. Serve with a green salad with oil and vinegar dressing.

Main meal
Any grilled fish with a green vegetable followed by some soft cheese with a large stick of crunchy celery.

WEDNESDAY

Breakfast
Half a grapefruit, 2 poached eggs, 2 grilled tomatoes.

Light meal
2 or 3 large flat mushrooms or a good handful of button
mushrooms fried very gently in a little butter in a covered
pan for about 15 minutes on wholemeal toast with a salad.

Main meal
Grilled lamb chops with most of the fat removed with peas
and carrots, a portion of dried fruits soaked and served
with low fat natural yogurt mixed with a pinch of cinnamon, grated lemon rind and a teaspoon of honey.

THURSDAY

Breakfast
A mixture of an orange, an apple and a pear sliced into a
bowl with a carton of natural yogurt and a teaspoonful of
honey.

Light meal
A sandwich of wholemeal bread without butter, a mashed
banana, a couple of chopped-up dates, a squeeze of lemon
juice and a sprinkle of any chopped nuts. A fresh pear and
a few grapes.

Main meal
Cut a medium-sized chicken breast into bite-size cubes
and marinate for 10 minutes in a mixture of half a
teaspoon of paprika, freshly ground black pepper, the
juice and grated rind of half a lemon, a tablespoon of olive
oil and a finely chopped clove of garlic. Remove the
chicken from the marinade with a slotted spoon, place in a
grill pan, baste with a little marinade and cook under a
hot grill, turning from time to time and basting again till
the chicken pieces are cooked through (10–12 minutes).
Serve with two different vegetables.

FRIDAY

Breakfast
2 boiled eggs, 2 slices of wholemeal toast spread very thinly with butter.

Light meal
A bowl of bean and barley soup (left over from Tuesday) with a wholemeal roll.

Main meal
Put a fillet of hake or cod on a finely chopped onion, tomato and garlic mixture onto a large piece of cooking foil, sprinkle more of the mixture on top of the fish, season with pepper and a little olive oil. Wrap the foil into a parcel, bake at 200°C/400°F/gas mark 6 for 20 minutes. Serve with a salad of watercress, orange segments and chicory. A piece of soft cheese (Brie, Camembert etc.) and a bunch of grapes.

SATURDAY

Breakfast
As much fresh fruit as you like.

Light meal
Italian toast – bruschetta. Toast a thick slice of coarse wholemeal bread until lightly brown on both sides. Rub one side with a cut clove of garlic, dribble on a little olive oil and pile with thin slices of fresh tomato – a wonderful snack for any time of the day or night.

Main meal
Chicken, beef or lamb casserole – remove skin and fat, cut into cubes, seal for a few seconds in hot oil, remove the

meat with a slotted spoon, add onion, garlic and celery, continue cooking till soft but not brown, add vegetable stock (from cube) with diced parsnip, carrot, swede, leek, turnip, potato. Return meat to the mixture, cover tightly and cook at 180°C/350°F/gas mark 4 for 1–1½ hours till meat is tender. 2 tangerines in segments with a small carton of fromage frais and a teaspoon of honey.

SUNDAY

Breakfast
2 slices of wholemeal toast with a little butter and honey. A glass of fresh orange juice.

Light meal
Green pasta and tuna fish. While the pasta is cooking put 4 coarsely chopped spring onions including the green tops into a frying pan with a little oil. When they're soft add a small can of drained tuna and stir until warm but not cooked. Drain the pasta, return to the saucepan, mix in the tuna and spring onions and serve. A piece of fresh fruit.

Main meal
Stir fry lamb. Remove all fat from the meat and cut into thin strips. Put in a shallow dish with 1 tablespoon olive oil, 2 teaspoons soya sauce, 1 tablespoon dry sherry and leave to marinate for 30 minutes. Then in a wok or thick-bottomed frying pan heat some olive oil, add the lamb and some of the marinade, stirring vigorously for 3 minutes. Add a small leek thinly sliced lengthways, stir for another 2 minutes, then add a chopped spring onion, a chopped clove of garlic and a little freshly grated ginger and cook for another 3 minutes. Serve with a tomato and onion salad. Half a small melon.

You must drink at least three pints of fluid each day – water, diluted unsweetened fruit juices and some tea and coffee. You may have one glass of wine or half a pint of beer or one pub measure of spirits each day as well. This is seven days of delicious healthy eating which I hope you will enjoy. It is not a diet but a guide to help you change the way you eat for the better.

CHAPTER 6

Sexercise

You are now in training for the Back Game and as with any sport you must get fit before you can really enjoy playing. Both men and women are just as likely to suffer an attack by the Back Brat and apart from the problems associated with pregnancy and osteoporosis in later life, the causes are just the same for either sex. In many ways women are at a greater disadvantage since they bear the brunt of caring for small children which involves lots of bending, lifting and carrying, and they often do most of the housework, the shopping, the cooking, the ironing besides often having a paid job as well.

Whatever your occupation – lawyer, dentist, builder, carpenter, lorry driver, hairdresser, bank clerk, computer operator, supermarket cashier or housewife and mother, you wouldn't expect to take up any sport today and be competing at international level tomorrow. And never forget that you are in double jeopardy – you've got a bad back and you're probably supremely unfit.

Sexercises will help solve both problems, your back pain and your generally low level of fitness. The two invariably go together – the back pain causes inactivity which causes loss of muscle tone, which causes back pain: a self-perpetuating cycle from which most sufferers can see no possible exit. There is one, but you must make the conscious decision to grab it with both hands and work at it. It is, after all, your back and your problem. Take the responsibility squarely on your own shoulders and do it now. No one else can do it for you. Be resolute, regular and responsible in your approach to sexercise and you will be rewarded with a level of sexual enjoyment that you have long believed impossible, and a degree of general health and fitness which dwindled away in your twenties.

Age is no barrier to sexercise, if you are twenty or seventy you can follow the programme to new vitality, new pleasures, and above all a new level of self-image based on improved energy and sense of well-being, better abilities in coping with stress, control of blood pressure, improved stamina, loss of weight and, of course, less back pain and a consistently high score in the Back Game.

Sexercise comes in two stages:

1. **Back to Basics** – Reconditioning the back and improv-ing posture, flexibility and strength.
2. **Fit for Bed** – A progressive sexercise plan for all-round health. Most people take to their bed when they are fit for nothing – you will go to bed fit for anything.

Some people are fiercely competitive and only enjoy exer-cise in gladiatorial atmosphere. These 'super achievers' make the fitness grade in combative sports. If you want to achieve physical fitness, follow the sexercise programme and avoid competition. The injury rate for competitive athletes is almost 100 per cent. Nearly all at some time suffer a stress-related injury which results in an enforced break from all exercise for a period of time.

Your only other competitor is the Back Brat, and you can beat him by guile, cunning and subtlety, not by hammering him to death on the squash or tennis court or running him into the ground in a marathon. If you enjoy games play them, but never lose sight of your prime target. The game is a means to an end. You gain nothing by over-extending yourself to win a tennis game only to scratch from the all-important Love Match. Use other games as the road to fitness, not the path to glorious victory and the osteopath. The only game you have to win is the Back Game and to do that you must prepare.

BACK TO BASICS

As any tennis coach or music teacher will tell you, practice makes perfect. There is no point in having a one-hour lesson each week and then ignoring all the good advice and instruction for the remaining six days and 23 hours.

You have to carry the lessons you have learned over into your normal life and make a superhuman effort to incorporate them into your everyday patterns of work, rest and play. Your body has developed its own habits, of posture and muscle tone and to overcome these handicaps you will have to make yourself constantly aware of how you sit, stand, move, work and exercise. By your own effort of conscious will you can superimpose new good habits over the old bad ones. If you do this often enough, the new patterns will become the norm for your body.

Posture is a full-time function and must be correctly maintained during every waking hour. Posture is also an outward portrayal of inner emotions and again the vicious circle of pain → inactivity → pain → depression is a vital contributor to your back problem.

You can put these problems out of your mind right now. No, that's not an idle promise but a guarantee. Most back sufferers, you included, can look forward to years of active living. You will have occasional episodes but you know how to cope with those. It won't be easy since you have to work, work and work again at making the postural changes you need. If you have the commitment and self-discipline you will make these changes. The leopard will change his spots and even the oldest dog can learn new tricks if the rewards are tempting enough. Your reward will be many years of happy fulfilment on the international circuits of the Back Game.

The ten times table that makes you able

Pick any ten of the following exercises and do them for one minute each *every* day and you will develop a new strength and mobility in your back which you never dreamed possible. Some exercises are compulsory, the rest are up to you. Just be sensible – more is not better. Any that hurt to do should be left for a while. You have to develop stamina and endurance and this takes time. You will soon learn to tell the difference between the acceptable fatigue of exceeding your own tolerance through hard work and the unacceptable fatigue caused by overstressing your already hard-pushed ligaments.

As your mobility and strength gradually return – together with your own self-confidence, you can progress to the more demanding exercises – but still only 10 × 1.

Three months of this simple regime will make you able to compete in the Back Game Championships, but remember that to achieve international status you then must move on to general fitness training. Before starting the Basic Back Builder's Programme, here are some fundamental exercises to get things moving and relieve the pain of acute episodes.

Low back stretching and postural exercises

Acute or chronic pain, injury, stress and muscle spasm can be the last straw initiating the vicious circle whereby a trigger point of fibrous tissue is created. This creates a continual irritant which in turn induces more pain and more muscle contraction.

The following stretching exercises are designed to

lengthen both muscles and ligaments, thereby breaking the cycle and changing the established behavioural patterns of the tissues involved. Before starting the exercises, you may find that application of ice-packs (frozen peas are ideal), gentle heat, or the alternate use of both, will induce relaxation of the tissues. This simple procedure usually makes the movements much easier and relieves acute pain.

This exercise should be done on the floor or a really firm surface. Bed is not the ideal place. All the lying exercises are best performed on the floor, preferably on a thin foam mat. Camping mattresses or sun bed covers are ideal and prevent pressure and bruising to the bony areas on the spine and sacrum.

Lie flat with a small cushion under the head, knees bent and feet flat on floor. Place hands behind thighs just below knees and *USING ARM MUSCLES* pull knees to chest and raise head. The pelvis must be raised off the floor. When you reach the limit of movement and comfort, hold the position for 15 seconds, then try to increase flexion gently. Do this in progressive steps for one minute.

After the exercise it is essential to lower *one leg at a time* slowly in order to maintain the gain in flexion and avoid the possibility of pain caused by a sudden return to an exaggerated hollow back.

Side bending – low back and shoulder muscles
This is done standing with feet 18″ apart and with slow deliberate easy movement. Five bends to the left followed by five to the right and holding each bend for 5 seconds. As you find the bends easier, you can bend the knee on the side to which you are moving. This increases the stretch imposed on the spinal muscles. During this exercise you MUST NOT allow your trunk to bend either forward or backward.

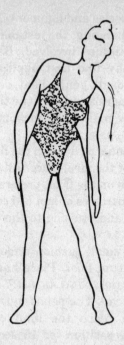

Tuck your tail in

Don't be a Back Bum. The Back Bum can be spotted everywhere and they come in all sizes and shapes, both sexes and any age. You can see them in bikinis, tight jeans, shorts, slacks, business suits, Dior dresses, maternity smocks, school uniform and workman's overalls. They all have one thing in common – backache.

The Back Bum can start in childhood, be caused by laziness or injury, occupation, or bad furniture or even be an outward sign of some psychological behaviour pattern. Whatever the cause, the end result is just the same. An exaggerated inward curve at the base of the spine (Lumbar Lordosis) and buttocks that stick out. The posture so popular with the advertising industry and used to sell everything from designer jeans to milk. The provocative sexual turn-on which looks great in commercials but is a

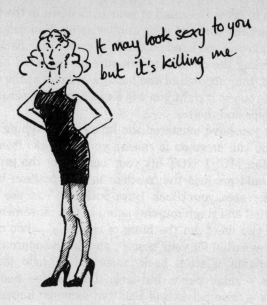

It may look sexy to you but it's killing me

real turn-off when it gives you backache.

This excessive lumbar curve distorts the entire spinal posture and creates pressure on the rear part of the lower spinal joints, squeezing the discs and nerves, and encouraging permanent changes in the muscle and ligament changes in the whole back structure.

Learning to 'tuck in' your tail means constant repetition of the exercises and concentration on your posture during all your waking hours. Persevere with these exercises and you will be firmly on your way to the championships and no longer a Back Bum.

The pelvic tilt
This exercise is suitable for all types of back pain, even acute disc pressure. This technique is most easily acquired lying flat on the back with both knees bent and feet flat on the floor. Place a small pillow under the head. The first

stage is to press the small of your back down to the floor, flattening the curve of your lumbar spine. You can practise by placing one hand on the floor under your back and then feeling the downward pressure on the hand as you contract your abdominal and buttock muscles at the same time. If you get it right you will feel a squeezing sensation in the hips and thighs.

Once you have mastered the knack of flattening your back you can move on to raising your buttocks from the floor. You MUST NOT lift your back from the ground. This would produce the 'restless bridge' position which only increases your Back Bum position. You use your abdominal and thigh muscles again in this movement.

Now you must get the hang of rhythmic pelvic movements, essential for your posture and for the approaching tournaments. Flatten back, raise pelvis, hold for ten seconds – relax pelvis but keep flat back – rest five seconds – raise pelvis and hold ten seconds. Repeat ten times. This exercise not only stretches the back muscles but increases strength and endurance in the abdominal and buttock muscles – so essential for tucking in the tail.

Now that you've mastered stages one and two you can start gradually straightening your legs, a little at a time, until you can perform the exercise easily with both legs straight out in front of you.

The standing tail tuck

Stand against a wall, feet about 6–9 inches away from the wall. Press the small of your back against the wall then slowly move your buttocks up the wall keeping your lower back in constant contact with it.

Now practise slow knee bends, keeping your low back firmly pressed to the wall and your tail tucked firmly in. This simple procedure strengthens the big muscle at the front of the thighs (essential for correct lifting) and teaches you to bend with your tail tucked in, thus

66

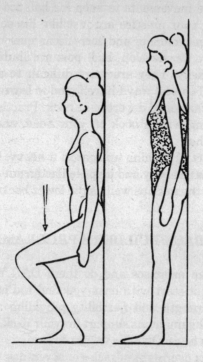

avoiding pain and unnecessary stress and, above all, this starts to improve your conception of upright posture.

Above all stand tall

Posture is a subconscious concept. We do not think about the muscles we use to maintain it or what they are doing from minute to minute. Why don't you fall over when you raise one arm to the side? Why don't you pitch face down in the dirt when you bend to weed your garden? How can you stand on one leg? All those are made possible by the 'synergistic' contraction and relaxation of your postural muscles, and you do not know a thing about it. Think of the high-wire man balancing with his long pole, making

67

endless minute movements to keep his balance 100 feet up in the air. Your muscles are just like his pole; thousands of tiny movements and corrections every minute. Unfortunately we develop bad postural habits very quickly and easily. They are more difficult to eradicate than acquire. The best way I have found to learn to stand tall is the old-fashioned deportment trick. Practise standing and walking with a book on your head, and a solid heavy one at that.

The mere fact of pushing up against a heavy, balanced weight realigns the body and helps to flatten out exaggerated curves in the neck as well as the lower back.

THE BASIC BACK BUILDER'S PROGRAMME

Choose any ten exercises and do them DAILY for ten minutes. Do not start with ones you find too hard. The objective is strength and flexibility providing all-round muscular and ligamentous support for your back. You are not training to be an Olympic weight-lifter.

Do not expect overnight miracles or seven-day wonders. You must aim at two or three months of relentless effort, but it will be an investment that pays huge dividends in the long run. Be prepared for occasional setbacks and episodes of back pain. Back pain is not a disease which will be cured like chicken pox or measles. It is a CONDITION mainly caused by wear and tear and you have to minimise its effects and maximise your own body's abilities to deal with them.

Never forget that hurt does not mean harm. There will be times when you decide that some pain is worth putting up with in order to enjoy a particular activity. If you follow the Back Builder's Programme faithfully, these occasions will become less and less frequent and the range of physical enjoyment that you find possible will get wider in time. This is especially true of sexual activity. You will learn how to avoid pain during the Love Game and minimise any discomfort that might occur after each match. Like any serious sportsman, your level of endurance and performance will grow with training and practice leading you to raise the level of your game beyond all expectations.

The 'flash in the pan' athlete who swings from rare flashes of brilliance to below average and dismal failure is no use to himself nor anyone else. Consistency is the name of this game. To scale the heights of regular, consistently supreme performance needs hard work and a real awareness of your own body. Ten minutes a day will set you on course, but don't give in and let the Back Brat get the better of you. Many of my patients get distressed and angry with their problems. My advice is always 'Don't get mad – get even' and your way to get even is to get FIT. Following these exercises will do just that.

Exercises

1. The tail tuck

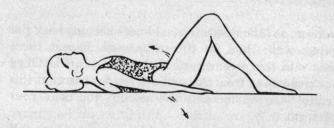

Position: Lying on back, knees bent, feet flat on floor.

Exercise: Flatten hollow of back on floor using abdominal muscles to pull abdomen down. Raise pelvis *just* off the floor. DO NOT lift lower back. HOLD for five seconds. Relax pelvis for five seconds but keep back flat on floor. Repeat five times keeping breathing regular throughout exercise.

2. *The straight leg tail tuck*
Position: as in (1).

Exercise: as in (1) but straighten legs gradually. This prepares you for exercise (3).

3. *The standing tail tuck*
Position: Stand with back against a suitable wall, feet 6 to 9 inches away from skirting.

Exercise: Flatten small of back against wall using abdominal muscles. DO NOT BEND KNEES. Hold for five seconds. Relax and repeat five times. Keep breathing. You can practise this exercise against an imaginary wall at any time when you are standing.

4. *The skier's tail tuck*
Position: as in (3).

Exercise: as (3) but slowly bend knees keeping back flat against wall. Hold for fifteen seconds. Repeat three times with five second rests. Do not let your flattened back come away from the wall. As you get better at this exercise you can increase the amount you bend your knees till they are at 90° – sitting on an imaginary chair. Carry on until you can hold this position for a full sixty seconds.

5. *The penny bum*
Position: Erect with a twopenny piece gripped between the cheeks of your buttocks.

Exercise: Flatten the lower part of your back and, keeping the coin held firmly in place, walk around the room for one minute.

6. Head up

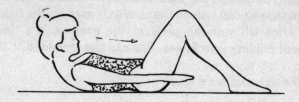

Position: On back, knees bent, feet flat on floor.

Exercise: Flatten back to floor. Arms up, chin on chest. Roll forward until shoulder blades are off the floor. Hold for five seconds. Roll back to floor. Keep tail tucked in. Build up to ten repetitions.

7. The sit down

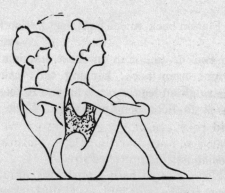

You must be proficient at this one before you can even consider the Sit Up.

Position: Sit on floor, knees bent, arms around knees.

Exercise: Lean slowly backwards, using your arms to support the weight of your trunk. Use your arm muscles to pull back into the sitting position. Rest for five seconds. Repeat ten times. As your abdominal muscles gain in strength, you can reduce the strength used by the hands and arms till you can perform the exercise ten times without holding your knees. You can then move on to (8).

8. The sit up with toe touch

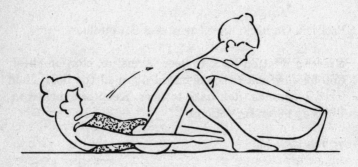

Position: Flat on back, knees bent, feet flat on floor.

Exercise: Tuck in tail, chin on chest, hands along sides. Roll upright from neck, keeping tail tucked. When upright, straighten legs, stretch fingers to toes, then roll slowly back to floor bending knees. Work up to ten repetitions.

9. The one hamstring protected stretch
Many athletes stretch both hamstrings simultaneously. Hamstrings are the large muscles at the back of the thigh. Loss of elasticity in these muscles inhibits lumbar flexion and correct spinal movement. Stretching both at once is

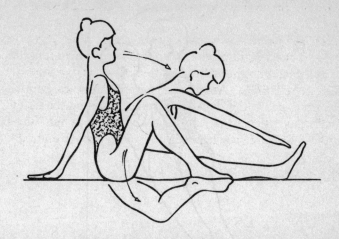

counterproductive since it can do harm and trigger pain without any appreciable benefit.

Position: Sitting on floor, bend one knee fully and place foot flat on floor. Allow bent knee to fall outward and stretch both hands towards foot of straight leg as far as comfortable. Now start a gentle rhythmic bouncing movement, reaching for the foot. Continue for twenty seconds. Rest, change legs and repeat.

10. *Away with Achilles heel*
Shortened Achilles tendons impede correct walking and limit knee flexion when bending and lifting. Consequently they play an important part in causing chronic back pain. These tendons may be stretched as part of number (9) by placing the foot of the straight leg flat against a wall and maintaining this contact during the exercise. Or do the following exercise.

Position: Stand 2–3 feet from a wall. Put arms out in front and lean palms of hands against wall, balanced on both

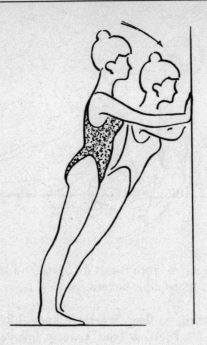

feet. Now place one foot halfway towards the wall. Keep other leg straight at the knee with heel flat on floor. Now bend the forward knee and both arms slowly and rhythmically. The back heel MUST be kept on the floor and the tail tucked in at all times. Continue for twenty seconds. Relax. Change legs and repeat.

11. The leg up
Lifting the weight of both legs off the floor together places a severe strain on the lower lumbar joints and unless you already have excellent muscle control, will inevitably increase the curve in your lower back. This most frequently induces pain. Until you are several weeks into your exercise plan just put the one leg up.

Position: Lie on back, one leg bent with foot on floor, other

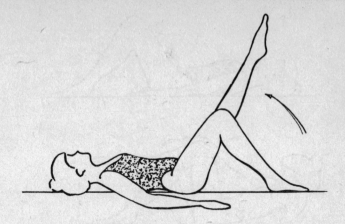

leg straight. Tuck tail in and maintain this position throughout this exercise.

Exercise: Without bending the knee of the straight leg, raise it upwards until it is level with the knee of the bent leg. Hold for five seconds, lower slowly, rest for five seconds. Repeat five times, change legs and do five more lifts with the other leg.

12. *Two legs up*
Position: Flat on floor with your heels resting on a chair seat. Your legs should be raised 30° at least. By starting in this position you avoid using the iliopsoas muscle and increasing your lumbar curve.

Exercise: Tuck tail in and maintain this position throughout the exercise. Keeping both knees straight, raise legs to 90°, and lower them slowly. Rest for five seconds and build up to ten repetitions.

13. *The crossover leg press*
This is an isometric exercise which really strengthens the abdominal muscles without movement. You are using the

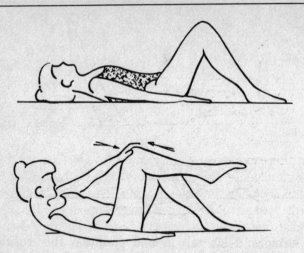

strength of two groups of muscles pitted against each other.

Position: Lie on back, knees bent and feet flat on floor.

Exercise: Tuck tail in and maintain this position throughout exercise. Raise right knee till calf is parallel with floor. Now place left hand on right knee, keeping your arm straight. Raise head and tuck chin into your chest. Now push hand against knee and knee against hand using the muscle strength of shoulder and arm against knee and hip. This creates powerful action of the abdominal muscles. Hold pressure for five seconds and relax.

Repeat five times then change over hand and leg, repeat five times also. Remember isometric exercise – NO movement.

14. The crossover sit up
Position: Flat on back, legs straight.

Exercise: Tuck in tail and maintain this position through-

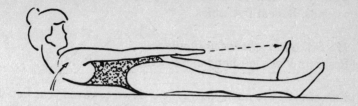

out this exercise, spread legs apart to 45°. Tuck chin into chest and place right arm across body. Now, pushing your right shoulder towards your left leg, raise your trunk until both shoulder blades are off the floor. Relax and repeat five times. Change arms and stretch left shoulder to right leg. Repeat five times.

These next six exercises are for strengthening and relaxing the neck muscles. Whether your original problem is at the top or bottom of your back makes no difference. The spine is one unit and although made up of many different parts, a problem with any section of the vertebral column affects the functioning of the entire unit.

15. *The chin up*
Position: Clasp fingers of both hands together and place them behind your head. Now try to lift your chin upwards, pushing hard against your hands. Maintain the pressure for ten seconds, repeat five times.

This is an isometric exercise and does not require any movement. Do not exert so much pressure that your neck muscles start to tremble since this will cause irritation of the muscle tissues.

16. *The chin down*
Position: Place the palms of both hands firmly against your forehead and press head against the hands, trying to

push your chin down towards your chest, hold for ten seconds. Repeat five times.

17. *Left and right ear to shoulder*
Position: Place left hand against left side of head.

Exercise: Try to push your left ear down towards your left shoulder, at the same time pushing with your hand against the side of your head. Hold for ten seconds. Repeat five times. Then repeat again with right hand on right side of head.

18. *The shoulder drop*
Raise shoulders as high as possible keeping arms by your side. Hold this position for five seconds then allow your shoulders to drop with their own weight. Repeat three times.

19. *Chest out*
Push both shoulders as far back as possible, sticking chest out and forcing shoulder blades together. Hold for five seconds. Relax and repeat three times.

20. *Chest in*
Push both shoulders as far forward as possible, narrowing chest and forcing shoulder blades as far apart as possible, keeping your arms by your sides. Hold for five seconds. Relax and repeat three times.

CHAPTER 7

Fit for Bed

Once you have really worked your back through the low back stretching and postural exercises, (see p62) you must build up a 10-minute routine of ten exercises chosen from them and the Basic Back Builder's programme (1–20). Three months of dedicated adherence to your chosen selection will do wonders for your back, but our sights are set on higher objectives. In order to make the World Rankings on the International Back Game Circuit, fitness is the prime requirement before you even consider the question of technique.

FITNESS

You may enjoy raising your 'fit for bed' factor in many ways and for a large number of people sport is an important factor in getting and keeping fit. Since you already have a back problem there are some sports which are not the most suitable. You may make a conscious decision to suffer some discomfort in order to enjoy your favourite sport. Provided that you are not in an acute stage of severe back pain, you will be better off enjoying an important cricket match and being uncomfortable for a few days afterwards, than staying at home getting more and more depressed.

I advise my back patients to avoid weight-lifting, judo, rowing, violent squash, contact sports, especially rugby, and above all jogging, since your feet hit the ground with all your body weight around one thousand times per mile. Swimming (not breast stroke), cycling, walking, ice or roller skating – providing you don't fall over – are all suitable.

Long-term fitness can be achieved by regular participation in aerobic exercise. That means continuous activity which maintains your heart rate at 75–80 per cent of the maximal rate for your age. This absolutely does not mean any of the fashionable aerobic classes. These classes are often run by untrained and unskilled teachers and can produce drastic problems for the fittest of participants, let alone you with your back. Aerobics classes are for staying fit, not getting fit, and even then they are the best thing that's happened to osteopaths since Prince Charles, and before him Stephen Ward and the Profumo Scandal. Now the latest craze of step aerobics is adding to the toll of back sufferers.

As if the 22 million sufferers of low back pain last year weren't bad enough, together with the 67 million working days lost to industry at a cost of £3 billion, we have an additional burden of thousands of self-inflicted back injuries as a result of step classes. These are often conducted in unsuitable premises, without the proper sprung flooring and by operators with insufficient knowledge of sports and fitness training. Few of those running classes are either aware of or inform participants of the risks of back pain, damage to the Achilles tendon, knee and ankle damage and overstretching of the joints between the bottom of the spine and pelvis. Many more people are purchasing step equipment for home use and suffering similar problems. Lack of attention to sufficient warming-up and warming-down exercises, failing to enquire about any previous history of back or joint problems and in some cases not even asking clients about high blood pressure, dizziness or heart conditions are all of great concern to the osteopathic profession.

Any continuous exercise which increases your breathing and heart rates is aerobic – walking, gardening, sawing logs or shovelling snow are all effective. You must aim at using 2,000 Kcal per week, which is the equivalent of three hours of sustained effort which maintains your heart rate at the required level for your age.

In order to avoid strain and damage it is vital that each period of exercise should comprise:

1. a warm-up phase
2. an endurance phase
3. a cooling-down phase.

The third or cooling-down phase is often omitted and is the reason that many people give up their exercise programme. Without it you do not encourage the elimination of waste products from the muscle tissues and consequently you are much more likely to suffer cramp, pain and stiffness in the forty-eight hours following exercise.

Recommended heart rates for best aerobic effort	
Age	*Heart rate per minute*
20	138–158
25	137–156
30	135–154
35	134–153
40	132–151
45	131–150
50	129–147
55	127–146
60	126–144
65	125–142
70	123–141
75	122–139
80	120–138
85	119–136

The fit for bed routine

1. **The Warm-up** This must last for at least five minutes, and is especially important if you have taken little or no exercise for years. The slow rhythmic stretching of the muscles increases the circulation and reduces the risk of muscular or ligamentous injury. You can choose any combination of the exercises 1 to 20, varying them from day to day.

2. **The Endurance Phase** This should last between twenty and thirty minutes so that you push your heart rate up to the appropriate speed for your age. DO NOT EXCEED THE RECOMMENDED FIGURE. Check your pulse rate a few times during the endurance phase. This is best done by stopping your activity and feeling the pulse in your temple with the pad of your third finger. Count the pulse of fifteen seconds and multiply by four to get the rate per minute.

   The objective is to speed up your breathing and heart rate without gasping for air. As you get fitter you will have to increase the intensity and the duration of exercise in order to maintain the required heart rate. If in the early stages of getting yourself fit for bed you cannot maintain vigorous exercise, you should do less intensive workouts but for longer periods of time.

3. **The Cooling-down Phase** This must last for at least six minutes and can include brisk walking for four minutes, alternate walk/jog for two minutes and any of the exercises 1–20.

   Work on the back exercises, persevere with the fit for bed routine and your partner won't know the vital, active and exciting new person in their life.

82

THE LOVE MATCH

In thirty-five years as a practising osteopath, hardly have a handful of patients with back problems ever mentioned their sexual difficulties to me straight out. Experience has taught me that any back conditions, chronic or acute, can and do affect the sexual activities of patients of both sexes.

Men, if anything, are likely to be even more troubled, since most women are more stoic and are prepared to suffer some discomfort. There is no doubt at all in my mind, that 'not tonight darling, my back is killing me' is rapidly replacing the time-honoured headache as the reason for saying no.

I usually have to broach the subject, and in a fairly light-hearted manner to avoid embarrassment – even in today's atmosphere of sexual equality and freedom, many people are not prepared to discuss their own particular problems.

'I should think your husband/wife is getting pretty fed up with your back problem by now?' normally brings the response: 'You know, I've been meaning to ask you about that. It is so painful that we've given up even trying to make love.'

Please do not give up. Of course, sex is not the only thing that matters in a good healthy relationship, but leave it out of the total male/female equation and you are asking for trouble. So many of the pinpricks and frustrations of daily life vanish in the comforting afterglow of loving and caring sexual activity, yet without it they grow and fester into seething discontent and disunity.

The Love Match is a game for two players, but it is not always essential that both participants take an active role in the proceedings. During the acute phase of an attack of back pain there is no reason why the fit partner should not provide sexual stimulation to their mate. It is true that the best lovers are unselfish. What better way to demonstrate your generosity than by helping your afflicted partner to an orgasm and giving them the pleasure as well as some benefit? The hormone release and increased circulation produced by sexual stimulation will help to relax their painful muscles and induce deep and restorative sleep.

The Ground Rules for this game are very, very simple:

1. Talk to your partner and establish what hurts, what helps, what positions they can or can't adopt and what they would like to try and what they wouldn't.
2. Take care to choose the best possible playing surface (see pages 48–50).
3. Never forget that above all sex is FUN. It is not something you do behind drawn curtains, in the dark, only because you want to 'have children. Whilst attempting to find comfortable positions to suit your particular back problem, you will have moments of pain and anguish which will be funny. Learn to laugh together, talk together and love together.
4. The objective of the Back Game is not to keep score, improve on your neighbour's performance, or keep up with what the latest magazine tells you is the national average. The ideal end is joy, pleasure for both partners, and a tender loving approach to each other's physical problems. The Ultimate Score is a DRAW where you each come out equal. If you achieve that, you've beaten the Back Brat and you're both Winners.

WHICH POSITION IS BEST?

As well as the sexual problems which are mentioned in my own consulting room, my postbag at the radio station LBC and from *Woman* magazine, where I write regular complementary health features, just goes to show that the few patients who consult me with sexual difficulties are just the tip of the iceberg. Backache in one or other, or sometimes both partners, is one of the commonest physical difficulties which interferes with an active and enjoyable sex life. Sometimes the problems are in the lower back, others have pain in the middle or even in the neck. Arthritis of the spine and of the hips is common and the lack of mobility which it causes can create difficulties as well as the pain. For example, a woman with arthritic hips finds it extremely difficult to lie on her back with her knees apart which makes the conventional missionary position about the worst possible for her. In the same way a man with severe lower back pain or with arthritis in his shoulders would find this conventional sexual position impossible.

For many couples, even after years of lovemaking, discussing the sexual act is still embarrassing. This is the greatest obstacle to overcoming the problem and leads to the route of least resistance – no sex. No matter what physical disabilities are involved, the giving and receiving of sexual pleasure is possible, even if normal intercourse is ruled out. Mutual masturbation and oral sex can both form a part of normal intimate relationships but when all else is impossible they at least provide an alternative to giving up sex altogether and enable a close, intimate and loving relationship to continue.

There are some positions for intercourse which place far less strain on the painful spinal areas and which are well worth exploring in the search for sexual fulfilment. It's no good just leaving this book lying around and hoping your partner will pick it up and be inspired. In spite of what you may hope, it is unlikely that your partner, however loving, will also be psychic. Having made one or two advances which are rebuffed because one of you fears the pain of continuing, most partners will give up. Don't let that happen to you. Talk about your problems, pains and fears and make experimenting part of the whole event of lovemaking. Keep your sense of humour because there will be times when things just don't work out and these are not the times to go off in a sulk, to feel rejected, inhibited or embarrassed. These are the times to have a good laugh together and remember the old proverb – if at first you don't succeed, try, try and try again. You'll be amazed at how much fun you'll have.

Some of these positions may not be the most romantic as you won't see each other's faces, you won't be able to kiss and whispering sweet nothings into your partner's ear is geographically rather difficult, but they do at least allow you to make love, and hopefully to find new ways of enjoying each other's bodies.

The missionary position in which you lie face to face with the man on top between the woman's legs is usually fine if it is the woman who has a lower back problem. In this case it is best not to use a soft bed but preferable to have two or three blankets or a duvet on the floor which will give more support to the lower spine. This does not work if there is a large weight difference, the man being very much heavier. This position is also good if the woman is suffering from neck problems, as long as there is one very thin pillow to support the head. This position is not good if it's the man who has the back problem, as it requires flexing and extending of the lower lumbar spine which can easily trigger muscle spasm.

This variation of the missionary position can be a great help if the woman has low back pain caused by an exaggerated curve at the bottom of the spine. By placing one or two pillows under the woman's buttocks, but not in the hollow of the spine, the pelvis is tilted upwards which flattens the exaggerated curve and relieves pressure on the nerve roots and surrounding muscles. As an added bonus this position can greatly increase the woman's sensations during intercourse.

If the woman has problems in the middle part of the spine, between the shoulders, a really good alternative is to start in the missionary position and then, in order to avoid the pressure of the man's weight on the upper part of her body, for the man to turn very gently through 90° so that he ends up lying completely across the woman's pelvic region, confining his weight to that area.

If the man has a lower back problem or the woman has a problem but her partner is much heavier than her, you can switch things around with the woman lying on top. This can either be with the man's legs together and the woman's legs on either side of them, or if the man's hips are not affected by pain or arthritis, with his legs spread apart and the woman can lie with her legs between them. This can be an extremely gentle and comfortable way of making love.

A variation of this last position is helpful if the woman has low back problems as it enables her to use her foot and leg muscles for movement rather than her back muscles. In this case the woman moves from lying between the man's outstretched legs so that her legs lie on top with the soles of her feet pressing onto the upper surface of her partner's feet. This can be improved even more if the man can have his feet against a firm surface and as few people these days have beds with sturdy footboards I suggest turning round in the bed so the man can have his feet against the wall or headboard. This avoids undue strain on his back muscles too.

Another good position when either partner or both have back problems is with her sitting astride him while he lies on his back. She should have her knees bent with her weight supported along her shins. The woman can then put her hands either on her partner's thighs or on his chest and use her thigh muscles to lift up and down. This avoids too much thrusting activity from the man and bending of the spine for the woman.

If the man has upper back or neck problems, it's good to start with the woman lying on top with her legs outside her partner's. She can then slowly lift one leg to the opposite side and twist her entire body until she is lying at right angles across the man – the exact reverse of the same position with the man on top. Whilst a little anti-social, this position can produce gratifying results.

Another position which can be just as good for the man or woman with back problems is for the woman to be on all fours on the bed with the man standing behind her at the foot of the bed. If either, or both of you, have back problems, this actually avoids flexing or extending of the lower back as the man can move by leaning forwards and backwards keeping his back straight and the woman can move simply by bending her knees. If the man does not have a back problem he can kneel on the bed behind the woman and bend his torso over her buttocks.

One of the most successful of all positions for any type of back problem is known as 'the spoons'. This is very comfortable and fairly effortless. To achieve the position the man lies behind the woman and if their relative sizes are suitable they can have intercourse in this position with the man achieving movement simply by rocking his pelvis backwards and forwards without using thrusting movements from the lower spine which would make his back pain worse. Where differences in height or girth make this difficult, either the woman can bend forwards or the man backwards, depending on whose back is best, and whilst not being quite so romantic as the whole bodies are not in contact, it's extremely effective.

Finally, if there is a history of either one of you having frequent back problems, the one item of furniture you should acquire is a sturdy, high-backed rocking chair. With the man sitting in the chair with his back and head fully supported, his partner can sit on his lap with her back towards him. Gentle rocking of the chair is all that's required, but watch out for the bare toes. If the woman's back is OK and she is fit and supple there are all sorts of variations on this position, which still leave the man sitting with his back supported.

GEORGE SEGAL'S STORY

Some years ago I was busy working in my surgery when the phone rang. It was an old friend saying that he was in the middle of shooting a film, they'd run into a problem and he was sending a car for me right away to come to the studio. Sure enough, ten minutes later, a limo arrived at my door and I was whisked away to the film set. When I arrived everyone was sitting around doing nothing, George Segal and Glenda Jackson were in bed and the director was stomping up and down shouting at everyone.

They were in the middle of filming *A Touch of Class* and they'd got to the scene where Segal finally persuades Glenda Jackson into his hotel bed and she realises one of her life's ambitions. No, it wasn't to have an amazing sexual encounter, but to see the sun rise over Gibraltar. In the midst of their lovemaking in the missionary position she looks over his shoulder out of the window and tells him that you can actually see the sun rise over Gibraltar. George was supposed to twist round to look out of the window and then get a spasm in his back. Unfortunately nobody on the set knew what would actually happen to him, or how he should act, which was why they sent for me.

George and I had a few quiet words and I showed him what would hurt and where and explained how excruciating and severe the pain would be if his back really did go into spasm. They cleared the set of everyone but the director, the camera and lighting men and me, and shot

89

the scene. His portrayal was so real and alarming that everyone else thought his back really had gone. But of course he's a brilliant actor and was only playing his part. Unfortunately for him he had a fall a couple of weeks later, hurt his back and did eventually end up on my couch for real. He turned out to be one of the nicest and funniest men I've ever met.

APHRODISIAC FOODS?

Where backache is a problem, you need to do as much as possible to encourage the gentle glow of romance which should be the beginning of all sexual foreplay. The heightened awareness, the tingle of anticipation and the excitement of sexual arousal all start the production of the brain's own pain-killing endorphins. Get the preliminaries right and the final outcome is much more likely to be a success. Often the key to the opening rounds of this game is the right food, the right drink and the right atmosphere.

Aphrodite was the Greek goddess of love and beauty, and it is from her name that we get the word 'aphrodisiac', which means, a drug or food which excites sexual desire. Our folklore is full of tales of these magic foods, but is there really any truth behind these old wives', or perhaps they should be old husbands', tales? Surprisingly, in spite of the fact that most people may scoff at the very notion of ordinary foods having such power, there is some scientific evidence that many of the traditionally sexy foods may actually help.

First and foremost, it is essential to understand that nutrition is the vital factor. The body has the amazing ability to switch off sexual function when there is more important work for it to do. During, and after, any serious illness, it is unlikely that a woman will menstruate, or that a man will produce sperm. The same is true in cases of severe nutritional deprivation, anorexics soon stop having periods, as do many serious women athletes. In order to enjoy a normal, healthy and satisfying sex life, the prime need is for a good, varied and balanced diet.

Assuming that this is the case, what then of all the stories about food to boost your desires, or your partner's performance? There is no doubt about the romance of eating. A candlelit dinner, 'à deux', is far more likely to end in consuming passion than fish and chips out of a newspaper on the kitchen table. Common sense should tell you that no man will be up to much after a meal of steak and kidney pudding, spotted dick and bread and cheese, all washed down with several pints of his favourite brew.

A light meal of subtle flavours, foods that provide the essential vitamins and minerals, blend wonderful colours and won't overload the digestive system, is what is called for. Do go easy on the booze. A little wine, or better still, champagne, will work wonders. But don't forget the infamous brewer's droop, or as Shakespeare warns more subtly in *Macbeth*, 'drink provokes the desire, but it takes away the performance'.

There are no magic foods or potions that will make up for a life of continual stress; that will compensate for a diet which does not provide enough protein, fats, carbohydrates, vitamins and minerals. On the other hand, there is no need for huge quantities of food, just look at the birth rates in some of the Third World countries. In fact, the opposite is true. Obesity is a common cause of impotence and lack of sex drive. This may be purely the result of psychological problems, or physical changes connected with being overweight. Chronic backache, or arthritic hips, do not make for good sexual performance.

There are many herbs which are reputed to have aphrodisiac properties. A mixture of rosemary and hibiscus is a simple favourite. Tea made of this combination certainly has a romantic and sensuous perfume. The ancient Greeks used the seeds of the ash tree which, they claimed, would 'render a man more spirited with the ladies'. The nasturtium, sometimes known as 'the flower of love', is not only delicious to eat, it cuts a romantic dash as a decoration on your dinner plate. And an infusion of the fresh leaves – half an ounce to a half-pint of boiling water – is thought to have a mild stimulating effect. In the Far East, the powerful properties of ginseng are legendary, in fact its common name is 'Man-Root'. One of the most famous of all sex books is the 16th-century *Perfumed Garden*. It advises men to eat strengthening foods like meat, eggs, aromatic herbs and sweetmeats made with honey.

From a scientific point of view, the most important nutritional substances for normal sexual function are zinc; the B vitamins, B6 in particular; vitamins E, C, and A; selenium and chromium. One of the richest sources of zinc is the oyster, one of the most popular of all the aphrodisiac foods. Casanova is said to have eaten at least fifty every day! Wheatgerm, oats, sesame and pumpkin seeds are also good sources of this vital substance. They are all rich in vitamin E as well, so it is hardly surprising that they too are part of the sex-food story. Beef, liver, the humble herring and eggs are other good sources of these vitality-boosting ingredients, all of which crop up in the folklore of romance and love. There does seem to be a need for some animal protein in the diet. A man's interest in sex may be reduced on a totally vegetarian diet, though the same thing does not seem to happen to women. From my experience with patients I think that it is the quality of diet which matters more. A bad meat-eater and a bad vegetarian will suffer in just the same way. Anyone who lives on burgers and beer, or white bread, pasta and puddings, is hardly going to make the world's most exciting lover. There is no doubt that a junk food diet high in the sweet and fatty foods will be low in those elements essential for all round good health.

Asparagus, figs, bananas, leeks, caviar, mushrooms and even hot spices are regarded as aphrodisiacs by some. And remember that chocolate contains both caffeine and theobromine. The former a stimulant, and the latter a chemical that gives feelings of euphoria and happiness, just like being in love. Why do you think that all those ads for chocolate are romantic, adventurous or outright suggestive?

Some of these effects are chemical, some mere folklore, some the result of our own romantic expectations. It does not matter which, if you believe in them, they will work for you. Curmonsky, who was Napoleon's personal chef, had strong views on aphrodisiacs and I'm sure that he was totally right when he proclaimed: 'Properly speaking, there are no aphrodisiacs capable of endowing those blind to life with sight. But for those with poor eyesight in this matter, there are substances which act as magnifying lenses.'

Intercourse is a simple physical act. Making love to a partner you care for is much more. The best aphrodisiac in the world is the touch or the cuddle of a loving, caring partner. Or perhaps those three little words . . . Mind My Back?

CHAPTER 8

Caring for Your Back at Work, Rest and Play

Let's take a look at how to avoid many of the common hazards that you will encounter at work, rest or play and that are a threat to your back. If you've never had a back problem there will be times when you look in the mirror and say 'Yuk!' There will be times when you dash for the bus and sit panting and sweating in your seat for the next twenty minutes. There will be times when the lift is out of order and by the time you get to the third floor you're looking for the oxygen cylinder. These are all times of danger because in a fit of enthusiasm you are likely to dash off and do the wrong thing. The trick is to get yourself fit for exercise before you start doing anything serious. If you really want to avoid damaging your back at the office, around the house, in the kitchen, in the garden, driving your lorry, standing in front of your class of children or tinkering with your car, then there are right and wrong ways of doing it all. The first bit of DIY on the agenda is to protect your back with a bit of general fitness.

Before you start pounding the streets, join the squash club or get out the aerobics books, make sure you won't be risking injury or putting too much strain on your heart. Because, although everyone knows exercise makes you fit, you also have to be fit to exercise. Remember the following golden rules:

● Make sure you're physically fit before you start.

Exercise can be enormously beneficial – it improves the efficiency of the heart and lungs, so helping protect you from future heart disease, chest and circulation problems. It helps dramatically with menstrual difficulties, is very effective in attacking depression and improves the body's overall resistance to infection.

But if you've ever had *any* chronic illness – particularly back or other joint problems, heart disease or high blood pressure – check with your doctor, osteopath or chiropractor before deciding which type of exercise to take up. Very few medical conditions demand a total ban on physical exertion, but some would preclude activities which might put strain on a part of your body which is damaged or at all vulnerable.

Your practitioner will also be able to advise you on what type of activity will actually be helpful in controlling your condition or promoting recovery. Those who have high blood pressure or heart disease, for example, would probably benefit from the relaxing effects of yoga, though they would not be advised to take up marathon running.

- If you're overweight, start with a non-weight-bearing exercise, such as swimming, cycling or just walking. Never take the lift when you can climb the stairs. Don't take the car or bus to the shops or office. Walking two miles a day and going up and down a few flights of stairs can easily burn up over 1,000 calories a week.

- If you haven't exercised for a while, don't start where you left off with strenuous activities. If you're going to an exercise class or gym, don't be too competitive in the early stages. Aerobics is great for keeping fit, but not for getting fit, so you should choose a gentler stretch and mobility class to start off with. Always warm up before exercise, and warm down afterwards. Aim for three sessions of physical activity a week, and make sure that you also exert yourself enough to get out of breath at least once a day.

- If you get a pain in your chest or feel dizzy, STOP immediately. If it happens more than once see your doctor.
- Don't exercise if you have a cold, flu or feel unwell. Your body has enough work to do fighting off the infections – it will need all the energy it can get if you're off colour.
- If you're over-35 don't take up squash – and don't continue playing unless you do so at least three times a week. Squash is the most demanding of sports – experts maintain that its erratic bursts of high activity put more strain on the heart and lungs than practically any other sport.
- Finally, but most importantly, you should enjoy what you do. Remember that nothing needs to be hell to be healthy.

Having got that out of the way it's time to consider specific activities and how to enjoy them safely.

LOOK AFTER YOUR BACK

At home

Homes can be decidedly user-*un*friendly when it comes to the back, so here are a few general tips. Do remember that it isn't only bending and lifting or even very heavy work that can trigger back pain. Awkward stretching and reaching up can be just as much of a problem. Combinations of bending and twisting or stretching and twisting can be fatal – not exactly life-threatening but a frequent trigger of acute back spasms. Silly things like stretching up and over an armchair to draw the curtains, bending at the waist and twisting to get something out of the cupboard under the sink, or even reaching across the table to pick up the pepper pot. You have to 'think back' constantly and ensure that you always move, lift and carry in straight lines. This is easy when your back hurts because it's the only way you can move, but the brain has an amazing ability to blot out the memories of pain. As soon as you feel better, you forget all about it and lapse back into your old bad habits.

The more you practise doing things the right way, the sooner good habits become ingrained in your subconscious memory and turn into automatic reflex movements. This requires constant vigilance and it helps a great deal if your family nag and shout whenever they see you doing things the wrong way.

If your backache is severe there are lots of useful implements that make life easier around the house and

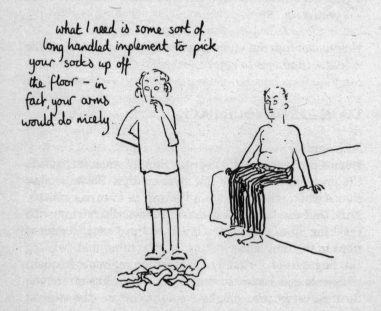

what I need is some sort of long handled implement to pick your socks up off the floor — in fact, your arms would do nicely.

one of the best is a 'third hand'. This is a long-handled grabber which enables you to pick objects down off shelves or up from the floor without having to stretch or bend. Larger chemists will have them or they're available from some mail order catalogues or through the Disabled Living Foundation (see reference section for address).

Your favourite armchair is not the place to sit and read a book or a newspaper, nor to write your Christmas thank-you letters with a notepad perched on your crossed knee – you should never sit with your knees crossed anyway as this rotates your pelvis, puts a strain on your lower lumbar and sacroiliac joints and is also a contributory factor in causing varicose veins. Sit up at the kitchen or dining table in a straight-backed chair. Support your book or writing paper on a sheet of plywood with 2″– 3″ blocks fixed along the edge furthest from you. This creates a gentle slope from back down to the front and means that you can read or write without bending your neck or leaning forward which puts a strain on your back.

You can purchase specially designed writing slides (address in reference section) which are portable and you can take from home to office if necessary. I'm certain that a lot of the increase in back problems starts in our schools. The old-fashioned sloping desk and bench or wooden chair have been replaced by flat tables and chairs which slope backwards so that they can all be stacked out of the way when classrooms are used for multipurpose activities. Children end up bent almost double at the waist, leaning on one elbow with their noses two inches from their books. This teaches them bad postural habits which stay with them for life. There's no doubt that the Victorians got it right in the first place.

Using one of Putnam's (address in reference section) wedge-shaped cushions is a huge improvement as you then sit with your thighs sloping slightly downwards, your back straight and in a much better position to read, write or play with your home computer.

Electric sockets are another bane of the bad back. Why builders insist on putting them in the skirting boards is beyond me. They're an ideal target for little fingers, and a nightmare for all back sufferers, and even more so for the elderly. When the time comes to have your wiring redone, shift all plugs to waist height and you'll be amazed at what a difference this makes to your back.

Make sure there is at least one sturdy upright chair with armrests for you to use somewhere in the house as you'll find that you place much less strain on the back if you can support some of the weight on the arms as you stand up or lower yourself into the chair. The Alexander Technique teaches us that putting your feet as far behind you as you can when sitting or standing enables you to move with the minimum amount of back bending and the least possible muscular effort. In this position most of the effort of raising and lowering the body in and out of the chair is performed by the thigh muscles.

Small children are another trial to the back sufferer and one of the commonest causes of acute back pain in new parents is dashing to the cot in the middle of the night. In your rush to pick up the baby before its third scream, you bend over the side of the cot and lever the bawling infant out at arm's length. A 12-pound baby held at arm's length exerts a pressure of sixty pounds on the base of your spine – that's more than half a hundredweight or a sack of potatoes. You must lower the side of the cot, squat down, gather the baby to your chest and stand up using your thigh muscles. This is true of all heavy objects which should be carried as close to the body as possible.

Don't walk around with your baby on one hip but use a baby sling, even indoors. Changing nappies with your baby on the bed is another sure way of aggravating your back. Obviously you don't want your pride and joy sliding off the draining board into the kitchen sink, but it is worth using a high trolley or stable kitchen table to do the job safely. Bending down to deal with toddlers is another hazard, especially for infant and playschool teachers. Again it's essential that you learn to squat with your back straight, but angled slightly forwards when dealing with them.

It may seem obvious but I'm always surprised at how few people think of even the simplest ways of avoiding unnecessary bending. They will happily fit a wire basket over the inside of the letterbox to stop the dog chewing up the bills but wouldn't dream of doing it to save them bending down to pick the mail off the floor. People go to endless lengths to stop the birds pecking the tops off the milk bottles, but do they fix a shelf by the door so that the milkman can leave them at a sensible height? Even when fitting locks or bolts to the front door the bottom ones are often almost at ground level. For security reasons they

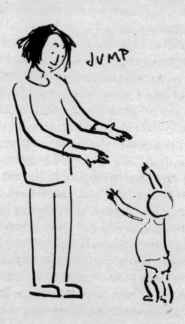

need to be as low as possible, but if they're so low that your back prevents you from using them they're not going to keep the burglars out anyway.

You must not be a martyr, nor must you worry about other people thinking you are a wimp. Taking sensible precautions will help prevent repeated episodes of back pain which is a pretty good idea as each time you upset your back it seems to happen more easily, the pain seems worse and the episodes seem to last for longer. Prevention is better than cure. Develop the habit of thinking about everything you do, making sure that you have the right tools for the job and planning your activities before you start.

JANET'S STORY

Janet was a typical example of how lack of thought can be a pain in the back. I hadn't seen her for about two years when she hobbled into the surgery. She had no idea of what had triggered this violent episode of low back pain and despite repeated questioning she couldn't think of anything that she'd done which could possibly be the cause. She'd learnt her lesson last time, or so she said. She was painfully getting dressed after the treatment when I asked her again whether she had done anything out of the ordinary. 'Nothing,' she said. 'All I did on Monday was wash the net curtains.' 'How many?' I asked. 'And how did you get them down and put them back up again?' It turned out that she'd taken the curtains down from five windows in the house and got them down and put them back up standing on a small footstool which meant she could just about reach the curtain rail if she stood on tiptoe and stretched to her full five feet four inches.

She was trying to save time by not going to the garage and getting the aluminium steps which would have been firstly, infinitely safer than a rickety stool, and secondly, would have enabled her to reach all the hooks without overstretching and all the subsequent pain.

Housework
It was Quentin Crisp who said that after three years of not doing any housework you stop noticing the dust and it never got any worse. Considering the problems that housework causes to back sufferers, I think that's a pretty good philosophy. Being clean is one thing, being a slavish, houseproud fanatic is another. It's really important to take care of the way in which you do various jobs around the house. You must also be realistic and just give up on those chores which really hurt your back. If you are a long-term sufferer then there is one basic rule which applies to housework, gardening and DIY activities, and that is – don't do the same job for too long at a time. Do a bit of hoovering, a bit of dusting, a bit of sweeping, a bit of polishing, then back to another bit of hoovering.

Don't stuff the vacuum cleaner into the very back of the hall cupboard so that you have to lift it over three pairs of wellies, two boxes of old newspapers that you've been meaning to take to the recycling centre for six months, a broom, a mop and a couple of buckets. I think that the suction cleaners with long handles and lightweight attachments are much easier to use, but they must have good castors on the main unit. Make sure that it also has a very long electric lead to avoid repeatedly plugging and unplugging. Ideally have two machines, one upstairs and one downstairs and if you can possibly afford it, get one of the very small hand-held cleaners for doing the stairs.

Forget about scrubbing brushes. You must not get down on all fours and scrub the kitchen floor from corner to corner. Use a long-handled squeegee mop and one of the non-rinse floor cleaning agents. Kneel to clean the bath and if you can't reach the other side, use your mop.

Kneel to tuck the sheets under the mattress and make sure you move the bed away from the wall rather than leaning over it. Better still use a duvet and fitted sheets. I never manage to get it right but I'm told that the best way to get the duvet into the cover is to push the duvet corner into one corner of the cover, hold the two together, push the opposite corner into the opposite corner of the cover, then, holding both corners of both duvet and cover, shake. If you can do it, you're very bright, or you've got very long arms.

If you've ever watched a professional roadsweeper, you'll have noticed that they never pull the broom towards them on one side of the body. They hold the broom in both hands in front of them and push in short strokes. Use this technique when sweeping and make sure you have a long-handled dustpan and a small, soft long-handled brush to sweep up the dirt.

One of the absolute no-no's as far as housework is concerned is window cleaning. The combination of stretching, pushing, and the circular movements involved are guaranteed to play havoc with an already damaged back. None of the 'easy to use' gadgets make any difference, as you always have to go round afterwards and get rid of the smear marks. Leave them dirty or pay a window cleaner every couple of months.

In the kitchen
Two domestic chores which are very common causes of back pain are preparing vegetables and ironing. Every patient I speak to says you can't do either of them sitting down, but you can. Sit at the kitchen table, peel and prepare your vegetables putting the vegetables in a colander and the peelings or waste on a sheet of newspaper. You can then wash the vegetables under the tap and put the waste on the compost heap. Most modern ironing boards have a height adjustment and by perching your

bottom on a stool with your feet on the ground to take the weight you can adjust the height of the board so that you can do your ironing with the least possible strain on your back. Have the unironed washing on a chair on one side of your stool and a convenient surface which you can reach without getting up or twisting where you can put the finished ironing.

As with television sets, most washing machines and tumble driers are too low down. If you can have them both raised about two feet from the ground that makes life much easier. Alternatively, use a stacking kit to mount one on top of the other and make sure you squat to fill the washing machine, don't just bend to one side and throw the washing in. Whatever you do, avoid huge piles of washing and ironing and try to do small amounts at a time. It may not be as energy-efficient as doing one large load, but what you spend on electricity will be more than offset by what you save on having treatment every time your back goes.

One of the great mysteries of life is why kitchen designers don't leave a footspace underneath kitchen sinks or work surfaces. If the base of your unit is level with the edge of the sink, your body is a foot away from the sink and three feet away from the taps. Back sufferers should always find a local carpenter who will remove the baseboard and, if necessary, cut out nine inches of the bottom shelf so that you can stand with your feet under the sink unit and your body right up against the edge. This avoids the perennial problem of being half bent over the sink and work surfaces when you're preparing food.

Floor-standing ovens are another great hazard. The door is inevitably hung the wrong way making access to the oven awkward and bending down to get a 20-lb Christmas turkey filled with 3 lbs of stuffing in a red hot dish swimming in gravy, 2 lb of roast potatoes and a pound of chipolatas is what makes most osteopaths busy on Boxing Day. Eye-level ovens and grills are safer, easier to clean and much less risk to your back. Heavy cast-iron cooking utensils may look great and be wonderful for making casseroles or omelettes, but they are not for the back sufferer. I'm not a fan of aluminium pans as there is still some question over the link between aluminium and Alzheimer's disease and some acid foods may dissolve traces of aluminium into the food. Although expensive, stainless steel is probably the best material as it lasts for ever and is easy to clean. Good quality non-stick pans also save a lot of hard scrubbing when it comes to the washing up.

In the bathroom
Finally, a few words about personal hygiene! Washing your hair, having a bath or cleaning your teeth can all be damaging to your health. The number of patients who end up on the floor with acute back pain after cleaning their teeth is quite alarming. Do not half bend over the wash basin but sit on a stool, squat or stand upright and use a plastic bowl to spit into. Don't bend over the bath or the washbasin to wash your hair, and be very careful getting in and out of the bath if you have a back problem. It's best to have proper grab rails professionally fitted, one that's at standing height and another just above the edge of the bath, so that you can get plenty of leverage and support. Grab rails that fit over the taps are also a good idea, as is a seat that fits over the edges of the bath and allows you to sit half immersed. This is an ideal position for washing the hair as you only have to bend your head backwards or forwards. For the chronic back sufferer, a separate shower is by far the best answer, but this too should have secure hand rails for adequate support. Always use a non-slip rubber mat inside the bath or shower and make sure that your towel is within easy reach when you get out.

In the garden

As you've already read, having a few different jobs on the go is the way to avoid putting strain on your back, whether gardening is a chore or your favourite hobby. Ten or fifteen minutes of each different activity prevents you being fixed in one position or from re-using one group of muscles for too long at a time.

There are a few simple things which make life much easier for your back in the garden. Lightweight, long-handled tools are a must, and it is really important that you keep warm. Wear several layers of clothing so that as you get warmer you can take one or two off, but do have a shirt or tee shirt long enough to tuck well into your waistband as the 'builder's bum' is a backache waiting for the icy wind. If you're digging, use a small spade or fork and keeping your back straight use the leverage of your knees and thighs to lift the soil. Don't dig for more than ten minutes at a time.

A lightweight wheelbarrow is another essential. Modern plastic ball barrows are very easy to manoeuvre but remember not to put hot ashes in them. Another alternative is a two-wheeled barrow though these can be quite expensive. Lightweight plastic sheets with grab handles are perfect for collecting leaves, weeds and prunings and they are easy to move around the garden. You can also buy plastic mesh containers with wire frames that stand up and open. A long-handled leaf grabber is another vital tool, but, better still, have a garden which only contains conifers.

If you're planning a new garden and you are a back sufferer, then go for large areas of patio, avoid vegetable gardens which need a great deal of work and concentrate on a low maintenance design which uses shrubs, ground cover plants and perennials so that you don't end up putting out summer bedding plants every year. A water garden is a good feature as they need little maintenance and provide a nice focus of interest. Avoid plants which need regular pruning like roses, and especially climbers and ramblers which can be a real problem because of the stretching involved.

Raised beds are the absolute ideal for anybody with a back problem, or for that matter with arthritis. These should not be more than four feet wide and around two foot six high. You can then do all the jobs without stretching more than two feet and with a minimum of bending. They can be constructed of old railway sleepers, stone or brick and though these are all quite expensive, they are permanent once they are installed. An alternative is to become a pot gardener with tubs, terracotta pots and other forms of container. Remember that once filled and watered, they can be very heavy, so make sure they're in the right place to start with.

Lawns are hazardous, though every English garden needs a bit of grass. Again, if you're starting from scratch there are slow-growing, low-maintenance grasses which need far less cutting and your local nursery or seedsman will be able to advise you. I don't think that the 'hover' type of mower is suitable for people with low back pain. The high-speed rotating blades always pull to one side and you need a constant counter-pressure in order to use these mowers. The best choice is a self-driven cylinder or rotary mower which you don't have to push. Electric ones tend to be lighter and you don't have the problem of pull-starting the engine. If your choice is a petrol mower, try to get one with an electric start, and if you have a large garden, a ride-on mower which doubles as a mini tractor to pull a trailer round the garden is a really great advantage. If you already have a pull-start mower, stand square on in front of the engine and pull the string with both hands straight towards you so that you don't produce a twisting and shearing strain on the lower part of your back.

The old gardeners say that the best time to weed is

when there aren't any, and they're absolutely right. Using a good quality, stainless steel hoe if you move gently between your plants regularly, the weeds will never get a chance to be established. This is exactly what you want as weeding a badly overgrown patch is almost certain to cause you twinges. If you have let things get out of hand, use your hoe and then lightly rake the weeds into a pile which you can pick up with your leaf grabber.

The new varieties of miniaturised fruit trees are a real boon to the back-disadvantaged gardener. They can be planted in the smallest of gardens, they produce crops on one or two stems and don't grow above a few feet, so that all the fruit is within easy reach.

If you have a greenhouse and enjoy doing your own cuttings or growing from seed, then it's a great help to fix the staging at the right height. Stand beside your work surface and measure about three inches below your elbow. This is the ideal height which you can work at without bending and you can relieve even more of the strain by finding an old stool and cutting the legs down so that it is exactly the right height for you to sit at and work comfortably at your bench.

Finally, a word about water. Carrying cans or standing for two hours with the hosepipe while you drench the garden should not be part of your plan. A small investment in trickle irrigation or a slightly larger one in a computerised, time-controlled, electronic watering system will pay handsome dividends. Not only will your garden look wonderful but you will be able to sit and enjoy it rather than being flat on your back at the height of the summer.

Gardening is a wonderful hobby and even with back problems you can continue to enjoy it providing you plan well, take extra precautions and restrain your wilder flights of fancy. The regular exercise of sensible gardening will help to develop and maintain mobility and muscle strength, both of which help to protect your back. Remember the parable of the tortoise and the hare. You only have to watch a real old-fashioned gardener and just as you think he's too slow to catch a cold, you realise than he can carry on plodding along for hours on end. You, on the other hand, go dashing out with your spade, attack the potato patch hammer and tongs and are indoors with a large whisky and soda nursing a backache after half an hour.

Travelling is a pain in the back

Travelling, actual or anticipated, is a common trigger of acute back pain which has ruined many a holiday or business trip. If you are a regular sufferer, travel as light as possible, preferably with a couple of small bags which you can carry in each hand rather than one large one which puts the strain all on the same side. Never carry a shoulder bag unless the strap is long enough to go over your head with the bag under one arm. Don't lift your own luggage in or out of the car boot, onto the weighing platform at the check-in desk, or off the carousel at the other end. Use a porter if you haven't got a strong-backed travelling companion – it's much cheaper than medical treatment when you arrive at your destination. Whether you're on a train or plane get up and move around as much as possible. Long flights in uncomfortable seats are dehydrating as well as a strain on your back. Drink a glass of water every half an hour, that will keep your body well hydrated and make sure you get plenty of exercise during the flight.

The worst thing about travelling is being late, stressed and rushed. Allow plenty of time for packing, preparing and getting to your departure point and try to have at least half a day off work the day before you travel. Mr. A. is a very high-powered international accountant and I know that when he hobbles into my consulting room bent over into a letter S and in violent pain that he is off on one of his regular trips to Australia and probably the next morning. He never allows enough time to finish off the work before he leaves, and consequently works himself into a state of frenzied tension trying to get everything done. The tension causes muscle spasm which in turn compresses the spinal discs pressing on the nerve roots and triggering the usual vicious circle. He never seems to learn but so far we've always managed to get him on the plane.

Finally, do wear loose clothing and your most comfortable shoes and never get onto the aeroplane with more than your ticket, your boarding pass, one good book and your essential toiletries. If you can't get it in the suitcase – don't take it with you, and more importantly, don't bring it home. Do you really need the half-size wicker donkey, fourteen bottles of that wonderful cheap plonk, three earthenware jugs and two armfuls of tropical flowers? You need them all like a pain in the back.

At the office
Stiff necks can be the result of injury, or disease, but they are usually caused by work, especially by office work. The stiff neck from which nearly everyone suffers at one time or another is nearly always due to muscle or ligament problems. Of course, bone, joint, nerve or muscle injuries or disease can be the underlying cause. But in the absence of any of these, muscular strain and fibrositis, nearly always related to work and posture, are almost certainly the reason.

When there is a physical cause such as whiplash injury after a car accident, or pain after any sort of fall, osteopathic treatment will provide the best relief in the shortest possible time. In the case of trauma this should not be undertaken before X-rays have been seen in case there are any fractures.

111

Repeated attacks of stiffness or pain may be directly associated with fibrositis, rheumatism, or arthritis, all of which in turn can develop as the result of bad posture. Where this is the case, there is no point seeking treatment unless you do something about the cause. Look at the postures you adopt at work. Is your chair sufficiently adjustable to support you at your desk or work station? Do you have a footrest or are your feet comfortably on the floor with your chair at the right height? Is the screen of your word processor at the right height for you, so that you do not have to bend your head forward or crane your neck upwards to see it? Is the screen offset to one side? Do you have a copy holder so that you are not constantly twisting your neck and bending forwards to read from papers at one side or other of the keyboard? Are you standing badly at your drawing board or work table?

It sometimes takes a considerable while to adjust your office chair so that it suits your particular size, build and shape, so be prepared to experiment until you find the ideal position. If you don't know how the adjustments on your chair work, then ask somebody who does. If you have to share your chair with other people it will probably need adjusting each time you use it, but if others only use it for a few minutes at a time don't allow them to change your settings. There is now a legal requirement for employers to provide proper chairs and work stations. If your chair is rickety, broken or the adjustments don't work, make a fuss. If you're in a union they will certainly take up these sort of complaints on your behalf and unions today are at the forefront of postural awareness. They will have experts who know all about the risks of bad office postures.

Your chair should be on a five-starred base and on smooth running castors. The back should be adjustable for both height and rake and ideally the seat squab should also be adjustable for rake. The whole seat must be adjustable for height and if it is fitted with armrests, they too should be height-adjustable to ensure that they fit under your desk top when necessary.

The advent of the word processor has caused serious problems for keyboard workers. Not only has it led to a dramatic increase in the condition known as RSI – Repetitive Strain Injury – but also it is responsible for more and more office workers suffering from upper back and neck strain. In the good old days of the typewriter you paused at the end of each line to push the carriage back; you stopped now and again to make a correction; you changed the paper, the carbon and the copy paper at the end of every page. Today a keyboard worker may sit for three or four hours at a stretch doing nothing but typing. No pauses, no breaks, no rest. This relentless repetitive work is what leads to the problems. No computer operator should spend more than a maximum of an hour at the keyboard without a break of at least five or ten minutes. After two hours there should be a break of at least half an hour when other jobs are undertaken.

Employers are none too keen on this idea but recent awards in the courts to people suffering from RSI may be enough to frighten them into submission. It must make more sense to look after the health of your staff than to have highly trained and key workers off sick for months on end.

Low back pain can also be a hazard in the office. The bottom drawers of filing cabinets should be kept for seldom needed papers. Photocopiers, fax machines and computer printers should be sited in accessible places which don't require the flexibility of a circus contortionist before you can change the paper, the toner cartridge or switch them on. No office worker should be required to move heavy pieces of equipment on their own and heavy boxes of office stationery should be delivered to the point of use by trolley or two strong men without back problems.

Planning the layout of your desk is a task which most office workers seem to ignore. You move to a new job, you take over somebody else's desk and leave everything where it was. It sometimes needs an element of detective work to track down this particular cause of problems.

BRENDA'S STORY

I first saw Brenda one snowy and bitterly cold February morning. Her boss was an old patient of mine and was most distressed to find his new receptionist sitting at her desk with tears streaming down her face halfway through her second week at his advertising agency. She'd developed dreadful pain in her neck, right shoulder, down her arm and into her fingers. She'd never had any problems before and she was convinced that she'd been struck with some horrible disease.

He put Brenda in his car and brought her straight round to see me. Brenda was an experienced receptionist/ telephonist and had always been very fit and healthy. She was only 28, played badminton regularly, walked a lot and went to a dance class at least once a week. I knew the office since her employer had asked my advice when completely refurbishing it a couple of years previously so there was no question of bad chairs, bad desks or bad equipment.

After some gentle stretching and massage the pain eased, Brenda realised that she wasn't going to end her days as a disabled wheelchair-bound old lady. She was certain that she'd done nothing to injure her neck so I sat her at my desk and asked her to rearrange everything on it so it was just like hers at work. Ten minutes later I went back into the room and found her sitting with the typewriter in the middle of the desk, the telephone on the left and her notepad and pencils on the right. I asked her to pick up the telephone and she stretched across with her right hand to the telephone on the left. She sat twisted in the chair with her right elbow balanced on the typewriter and her neck turned almost as far to the left as it would go.

The previous receptionist had been left-handed! I moved the telephone to the other side of the typewriter and told her to try again. Abracadabra – a wave of the old magic wand – a sprinkle of the stardust and the problem was solved. To the best of my knowledge she's still in the same job five years later, and I haven't seen her since.

SELF HELP

The very nature of office work is sedentary and to compensate for this you should make sure that you are physically active in your leisure time. It's extremely important to try and maintain the maximum possible movement in all the joints and muscles of the neck, so try these simple exercises. They are not physical jerks and should be done slowly and gently and repeated frequently during the day.

Sit in an upright chair, clasp your hands together and place them on the back of the head. Now drop your chin forward onto your chest, don't pull with your hands, just let the extra weight of your arms stretch your muscles a little further than they would go on their own.

Place your right hand on top of your head with the fingers just above the left ear and use the arm to pull your right ear towards your shoulder. Do this several times, feeling the muscles stretch as you do it. Move your right hand to your chin and turn your head to the left using the hand to push your chin towards your left shoulder.

Change hands and repeat both exercises. Finally, drop your chin onto your chest and very slowly roll your head in a circle, stretching it as far as you can in every direction. When your chin ends up back on your chest, repeat in the opposite direction.

You can get great relief for your stiff neck by applying alternate hot and cold compresses to the back of the neck and shoulders. You should leave the hot compress on for two minutes, but a cold one for about ten seconds. This helps to stimulate the circulation and disperse the build-up of lactic acid produced by tense muscles.

Any form of gentle massage will help, especially if you use one of the specific herbal oils for the relief of muscular pain. The best of these is Flexarome, made by the famous French herbalist Dr. Jean Valnet, and available from good health stores.

The neck and shoulders are the most common site for stress-related muscle tension, and, of course, the trigger point for headaches. If you suffer repeated or continual discomfort you really need to get some help in order to break the vicious circle of stress, muscle tension, pain, and more stress. See your local qualified osteopath or chiropractor as soon as possible.

Your best protection is your common sense. With any physical activity the key to success is little and often combined with variety of movement. Know your own limitations – it's no good spending all day painting skirting boards or sanding down the wooden floor or painting five ceilings if you've got a back problem. You will never succeed in laying fifty square yards of crazy paving, or wheelbarrowing five cubic yards of concrete from front drive to the back garden. Your back won't enjoy pulling a heavy roller over the lawn, or spending all day spiking it. Your painful neck will suffer if you spend all day screwing in new curtain rails with your head squashed against the ceiling. You certainly won't survive hanging kitchen cupboards on your own, wedging them with one knee halfway up a ladder and driving in four-inch screws with one hand.

It's not all gloom and doom. Hurt is not the same as harm and if you enjoy a bit of woodwork, building a brick wall, cooking a gourmet meal or polishing the family silver, you won't do any damage as long as you're sensible. Yes, it may hurt a bit when you've finished, but if the satisfaction of a job well done and the enjoyment of completing a task which gives you pleasure is what you want, then carry on. With a bit of care, a lot of enthusiasm and a pinch of perseverance you'll be Back to Strength in no time.

CHAPTER 9

The Full Treatment

It is necessary to know the spine and what its natural purposes are, for such a knowledge will be requisite for many diseases. (Hippocrates)

As you've already read in Chapter 1, many people with back problems have at best a sketchy knowledge or at worst a depressingly wrong picture of the causes and treatments of back pain. Not long ago all unorthodox treatments were thought of as 'fringe medicine'. But happily modern trends are moving towards much closer cooperation between the orthodox and the complementary practitioners of the healing arts. And complementary is the correct word to use. There is no such thing as alternative medicine, there is only good medicine and bad medicine, and that – sad to say – is practised on both sides of the fence. There are some conditions which are best treated by complementary medicine. There are some best treated by the orthodox. But the vast majority of patients get the best of both worlds when the treatment is truly complementary – each branch of medicine contributing its own special skills.

In the case of back problems this is even more true and the growing collaboration between osteopaths, chiropractors and orthopaedic surgeons is leading to greatly improved treatment for the long-suffering patients. We've already seen the passage of the Osteopath's Bill through Parliament which will lead to a

Statutory Register. Chiropractors, acupuncturists and others will follow. A number of the leading training schools are now able to award recognised BSc degrees to their graduates and all in all, it is getting easier by the day for the general public and the medical profession to identify the bona fide complementary practitioners. In order to help you help yourself to a better back, let's look at what the different therapies have to offer.

OSTEOPATHY

Osteopathy is a system of healing primarily concerned with the structure and correct alignment of the body and thus the body's function. The bones, joints, ligaments, tendons, muscles and general connective tissue, and, most importantly, their inter-relationship, comprise the body's musculo-skeletal system. Many osteopaths believe that the body will keep healthy provided there are no structural defects, such as a displaced bone or vertebra, and these can be corrected by manipulation. These musculo-skeletal defects are thought to affect local nerves, and, therefore, because the nervous system functions as a whole, defects will adversely affect the organs of the body, all of which are controlled by the nervous system. Once the defects are corrected, one can reasonably expect the benefits to be transmitted throughout the nervous system and thus to the organs of the body.

What is osteopathy?
The term osteopathy was first used by its founder, Dr. Andrew Taylor Still (1828–1912) of Missouri, in 1874. He believed that the human body was self-healing and that an uninterrupted nerve and blood supply to all the tissues of the body was indispensable to their normal function. If any structural problems, such as curvature of the spine,

interfered with this nerve and blood flow, the self-healing power was disrupted and disease would result. With this in mind, Still worked out a system of manipulation intended to realign any structural deviations or abnormalities.

Manipulation of the musculo-skeletal structure has a long history. Until Still's time, however, spinal manipulation was used solely to treat conditions of the back at least in Western orthodox medicine. Still extended the use of manipulation to cover the treatment of the whole body, adopting many of those techniques that were valuable and rejecting those that were of no use or possibly even dangerous, to create a complete and practical therapy in which structure and function of the body are seen to be completely dependent on one another. In 1892, Still founded the first school of osteopathy, in Missouri. One of his students, John Martin Littlejohn, who had earlier studied physiology for three years at Glasgow, founded the British School of Osteopathy in 1917 a few years after his return from the United States.

How can it help?
Most people who consult an osteopath for the first time are usually suffering from back problems or pain and discomfort in other joints and muscles. It is not unusual, however, to find that after treatment for the main complaint, patients also report improvements in other conditions which they did not think suitable for osteopathic treatment. For example, the patient suffering from neck and shoulder pain and stiffness may find that manipulation of the vertebrae in the neck has also relieved dizziness or headache.

Modern research in American osteopathic hospitals has shown how abnormalities of the spinal column can affect organs such as the lungs, heart, stomach, intestines, bladder and uterus. It can also be demonstrated that these organs can affect the spine. Manipulation, therefore, can be shown to be of great value in the treatment of many conditions, especially migraine, asthma, constipation, menstrual pains, heart disease and digestive disorders.

Osteopaths do not consider the spine to be the only factor in the cause of disease; illness can be caused by genetic factors, dietary, environmental, psychological and bacterial influences. While osteopathic treatment may relieve some of the symptoms of these problems, it cannot claim to cure diseases of this nature.

How does the osteopath work?
The osteopath examines the patient from the moment he/she enters the consulting room:

- How do they walk?
- How is their posture?
- How are their movements?
- Are they stiff and rigid?
- Are they bent at the waist?
- Is their back out of alignment?
- How do they sit in the chair?

All these things are vital clues to the origin of the patient's problem. Before an osteopath treats a patient for the first time, he or she takes a detailed medical history. This is followed by a complete physical examination in which the osteopath will examine posture and the way in which the patient moves, and will observe restrictions or exaggerations of movement in any area of the spine. Then a detailed examination of the spinal column follows, testing the movement of each vertebra, looking for tenderness, stiffness or displacement. Further tests, such as X-rays or blood or urine analysis may be recommended to help reach an accurate diagnosis.

Assuming that osteopathic treatment is appropriate to the condition and that there are no contra-indications to manipulative treatment, the osteopath sets out to improve the mobility of impaired joints, restoring function to those which are not working properly and relieving areas of pressure (which may be affecting those nerves supplying very distant parts of the body) by manipulating the patient's back, limbs, or other joints. The osteopath may use techniques of manipulation, deep neuromuscular massage along the nerve routes, relaxation and postural re-education, all with the object of relieving the cause of the patient's condition. It is not uncommon for patients to suffer some form of reaction, such as the aggravation of existing symptoms or discomfort in the treated area, after the first one or two osteopathic treatments since the manipulative thrust which is used to readjust the spinal joint can sometimes irritate the surrounding tissues.

Patients often expect the osteopath not to be in favour of the use of drugs or surgery for the treatment of back problems and this in broad principle is true. There are situations, however, when anti-inflammatory drugs, preferably non-steroidal, or pain-killers should be recommended for brief periods at times of acute pain. There are a few situations in which spinal surgery is inevitable but osteopaths believe that many people submit to it before exploring all the alternative possibilities of manipulative treatment. More and more orthopaedic surgeons are recommending their patients to try osteopathic treatment, if other orthodox forms have failed, before resorting to spinal surgery. This complementary use of the skills of the orthodox orthopaedic surgeon and the osteopath is undoubtedly in the best interest of the patient and produces results which in some instances neither practitioner could achieve alone.

Back matters

It is the holistic approach taken by the osteopath that accounts for the high success rate in the treatment of back problems. Many patients who have suffered back problems for years have never had a thorough spinal examination. The visit to the osteopath is often the first time the back sufferer has been asked to take his clothes off. Yet it is quite impossible to arrive at any diagnosis of a back problem without examining the patient standing, sitting, lying and moving without clothes on, feeling the skin and muscle tone and establishing an understanding of the integrity of the underlying structures.

An osteopath looks at the patient as a whole entity. Although back pain may be the symptom with which the patient presents himself in the osteopath's surgery, the root cause of that pain can be far removed from the back itself. Simple problems with the feet, ankles, knees or hips can frequently result in back pain. Changing the height of the chair in which the patient works, altering the height of the bench in the factory or workshop or merely changing the type of shoes he wears can dramatically improve long-standing and chronic back problems.

Cranial osteopathy

Cranial osteopathy is a specialised technique described as 'indirect' as no manipulative thrust is applied to any spinal joint. The cranial osteopath believes that the fine joints, or sutures, of the bones that form the skull allow tiny movements to occur between them. By stimulating this movement, the circulation of cerebro-spinal fluid is encouraged which may relieve local symptoms and also affect other organs, such as the pituitary gland. This technique can be especially helpful in the treatment of children with learning difficulties and those with some forms of brain damage. Gentle, rhythmic pressure is applied to the head in order to encourage movement of the skull sutures.

CHIROPRACTIC

This is a form of manipulative treatment closely aligned to osteopathy. The concept of chiropractic (it means treatment by the hands, or manipulation) was developed by David Daniel Palmer (1845–1913) in 1895 in Iowa. He believed, like Still, that displacements of the structure of the spine cause pressure on the nerves which in turn cause symptoms in other parts of the body. The main differences between chiropractic and osteopathy are mostly historical since both forms of manipulative therapy now subscribe to the modern concepts of anatomy and physiology, although they both use manipulative treatment for the relief of a wide range of disorders rather than just disorders of the spine. Like the osteopath, the chiropractor considers the patient as a whole, with the emphasis on the body's structure, in relation to the patient's specific problem.

The chiropractor tends to place a greater reliance on X-rays in the diagnosis of spinal problems than the osteopath and the techniques of manipulation are slightly different to those of the osteopath. The chiropractor tends to use less leverage and more direct thrust against the specific vertebrae. Chiropractic treatment can achieve excellent results in the treatment of back pain, other musculo-skeletal disorders and certain systemic disease, such as asthma, migraine, digestive and menstrual disorders.

In Australia and the USA, the chiropractor has the same status as osteopaths do in Great Britain since they remain outside the realms of orthodox medicine. Like the British osteopaths, there are many British practitioners calling themselves chiropractors but far fewer who belong to the established chiropractic association. There are more osteopaths than chiropractors in the United Kingdom, although the establishment of the excellent Anglo-European College of Chiropractic has led to a growing number of highly qualified practitioners. In Australia there are more chiropractors than osteopaths. The regulations and practice vary from state to state both for chiropractors and osteopaths. (See Appendix for details of professional bodies for all three countries.)

MASSAGE

The ancient art of massage is both luxurious and relaxing and, in the context of natural health, the most innocuous of all the therapies. A good massage can soothe headache, relieve tension and stress in the body, help insomnia, relax taut muscles, lower the blood pressure and, above all, induce a feeling of calm, suppleness and well-being. It is well worth taking massage as a regular basis for relaxation and as a preventative treatment for stress.

How massage works
Massage concentrates on the soft tissues of the body, the muscles and ligaments, in order to stimulate the circulation of the blood and the functioning of the nervous system. At the same time, the blood pressure is lowered as a consequence of the soothing movements.

Footballers, athletes and dancers find massage particularly beneficial as it negates the unpleasant side-effects of hard exercise and prevents the muscles becoming too taut. During exercise, waste products are released into the muscles and these wastes are later drained away by the lymphatic system. This process can take up to several days, and the accumulation of waste products is what causes stiffness after exercise. Massage speeds up the draining process by stimulating the lymphatic system and the circulation of the blood. Massage is also a useful adjunct to physiotherapy and manipulative therapies.

Types of massage
There are two principal systems of massage: **Swedish massage**, which is the system used chiefly in the West, and **Shiatsu massage**, from Japan, which combines massage with acupressure on the body's meridian system and acupuncture points.

Swedish massage
Swedish massage relies on the four basic techniques of *effleurage, pétrissage, pressure* and *percussion* carried out in turn on the back, arms and hands, abdomen, feet and legs, head and face. The most important point to remember in mastering the techniques is that contact with the body should not be broken. The ideal is to create a rhythmic and continual movement, with the techniques producing an alternating soothing and stimulating effect.

Effleurage
This is a rhythmic stroking movement with open relaxed hands, designed to soothe and relax the body and to maintain a rhythm throughout the massage so that one movement flows into another. Effleurge movements are also directed towards the heart, while stroking can take any direction.

Pétrissage
This is an intermittent deep movement of lifting, rolling, pressing or squeezing, not unlike kneading bread.

It is designed to stimulate the muscles and areas of fatty tissue. It stretches those muscles that have seized up and become shortened and relaxes contracted muscles.

Pressure
The third technique is designed to set up friction in order to stimulate the body's superficial tissues. Small circular movements are made with the thumbs, fingertips or heel of the hand. Pressure is exerted before each circular movement and, during the movement, the skin moves under pressure from the fingertips against the underlying body structure. It is designed to relieve specific areas of tension, such as around the neck, shoulders and buttocks.

Percussion
Percussive movements are the most difficult for the non-professional to perfect: they are brief, brisk, rhythmic, springy movements applied in series with alternate hands. They consist of cupping, hacking, flicking, pummelling and clapping movements in order to stimulate the skin and, in turn, the blood circulation. These are followed with effleurage in order to soothe and to maintain a rhythmic contact with the body.

Although massage is for the most part beneficial, remember that you must not have a massage if you are suffering from any of the following:

- any infectious, erupting skin complaint
- large bruises
- varicose veins
- temperature/fever
- inflamed joints or are at the acute stage of arthritis
- thrombosis or phlebitis as a blood clot could be disturbed.

AROMATHERAPY

'The way to health is to have an aromatic bath and scented massage every day . . .' declared Hippocrates many centuries ago. Certainly, the use of aromatic oils greatly enhances a massage treatment, turning it into a positively pampering experience. Using essential oils during massage to treat specific disorders is known as aromatherapy, a technique based partly on the fact that different smells produce different emotional reactions and partly on the individual properties of essential oils which may exert a therapeutic effect on the body. Recent research at Kneipp Institute in Germany has demonstrated that the essential oils are absorbed by the skin, enter the bloodstream and can be measured in the exhaled breath, having done their therapeutic job on the way.

Concentrated essential oils can cause stinging and allergic reactions, so just one or two drops of essential oil to every 5ml (1 teaspoon) of 'carrier' vegetable oil is sufficient. The masseur applies a little of the oil to his/her palms and applies it to the body in one long stroke.

Types of essential oils
The essential oils are used either singly or as a mixture. In perfumery, scents fall into three categories, depending on their rate of evaporation: top, middle or base notes. The top note makes the initial impact, the middle note provides the mellow note and the base note is long-lasting.

THE ALEXANDER TECHNIQUE

The Alexander Technique is a process of physical re-training that has far-reaching positive effects on both mental and physical health. The human body is a complex, delicately balanced piece of engineering. Muscles and bones are designed to interact harmoniously in such a way as to enable us to walk and move with maximum ease and minimum strain. All of us are born with a natural ability to use our bodies the way they were intended, but from a very young age most people start to misuse them, developing mannerisms that throw the whole body out of true; slouching at the desk at school; stiffening unnaturally straight for gym. Constant repetition makes these bad physical habits feel 'right' and we lose our inborn instinct to return to correct, healthy posture. The result of misuse is a malfunctioning of our whole system. The Alexander Technique aims to help you relearn the correct way to use your body by substituting a set of positive habits for the bad ones, so that gradually you become aware of your body's misuse and are able to correct it by returning to a better use of self.

How the Alexander Technique works

The Alexander teacher conveys the technique by gently realigning and manipulating the student's body. As he or she works they will repeat certain key phrases, such as 'neck free, to allow the head forward and up, back to lengthen and widen'. Through repetition the student comes to recognise the feeling of correct use and connects this with the corresponding phrases, or 'directions'. In everyday life they will soon be able to feel when they are slipping into bad use, and 'come back to their directions'. The key is the relationship between the head, neck and back. The head is very heavy, so needs to be properly balanced. Thrown back or tipped too far forward – the two most common misuses – the muscles of the neck strain to hold this heavy object, creating tension, and limiting the 'free' movement of the head. The spine, too, is often contracted or thrown out of shape by misuse which means it is impossible to use the rest of the body correctly.

The Alexander teacher also concentrates on correcting *endgaining* – the common habit of striving too hard to do something so that you tense your muscles at the very thought of what you have to do. You might, for example, grip a pen too tightly. It is comparable with the energy and force you expend when you pick up an empty suitcase, thinking it is full. Learning to inhibit this instinctive reaction allows you correct control.

Alexander lessons

Alexander lessons are given on a one-to-one basis. Because your own ingrained habits have come to feel so comfortable, it is impossible to correct your *endgaining* yourself: the theory is not enough to convey the technique. The teacher shows by gentle manipulation and the explanatory 'directions' how proper use should feel. The adjustments are small and subtle. There is no wrenching or forceful realigning. As some wrongly used muscles must learn to lengthen, and other under-used muscles must start to work, the technique coaxes rather than pushes to allow the body to come into a more balanced position.

Teachers apply the technique in their own ways. But each teacher's method hardly varies from lesson to lesson. The student is shown correct use in the basic positions of sitting, standing and lying down. The technique of getting in and out of a chair is included in each lesson, because it is something we do many times every day – and it demonstrates our misuse in movement. The repetition of exactly the same movements and positions in each lesson serves to create the necessary new habits and awareness.

The hardest thing for a student to learn initially is not to interfere, 'non-doing'. When the teacher lifts your arm or guides you into a sitting position, it is automatic to give some help with your own muscular effort. Learning to inhibit these unconscious muscular movements is an important first step towards correct conscious control. But all students report an extraordinary feeling once the teacher has moved them into the perfect balanced position. There is a general feeling of well-being, a lightness and an exhilaration.

Each lesson lasts for half to three-quarters of an hour. It is usually recommended that new students have lessons three times a week for the first few weeks; after that, once a week is enough. An average of thirty lessons is considered sufficient to re-educate yourself to the point where you can carry it on into daily life, though some people choose to continue for many years, returning periodically for reminders.

Doing it yourself

Although you cannot learn the technique without a student/teacher relationship, the whole aim of the teaching is to enable you to carry out the technique in your everyday life. Some teachers recommend that you practise the 'lying down' as taught, for fifteen minutes or so a day. This position, with your head slightly raised by a book, and your knees bent, puts your spine in its correct, lengthened position.

How can it help?

The Alexander Technique has a beneficial effect on any number of physical problems, including hypertension, asthma, peptic ulcers, spastic colon, ulcerated colitis, rheumatoid arthritis, tension headaches and low back pain. The positive health benefits in improved performance are recognised by athletes and major drama and music colleges, which have resident Alexander teachers. (Alexander was himself an actor.)

The technique has a positive effect on the general functioning of the body, especially the circulation of the blood and breathing. It is enormously beneficial in dealing with stress. Muscle tension is fed back to the brain as feelings of stress and panic. Relaxation techniques usually only help for the period that they are being used, whereas the Alexander awareness will enable you to recognise whenever a muscle in any part of your body tenses up, and therefore to release it and prevent stress build-up.

RELAX AWAY YOUR BACKACHE

Stress and tension are both cause and effect in many back sufferers. Postural tension brought on by bad office seating, poorly designed work stations and repetitive muscular effort in awkward positions – ask any VDU operator, supermarket checkout operator, assembly line worker, plumber or garage mechanic – is one of the commonest causes of stress-induced back pain. On the other hand, anyone with arthritis of the spine, a chronic disc problem or injury-induced back pain will inevitably become tense as a result of the discomfort, the inability to perform and the frustration of leading a restricted life.

Either way, the stress causes muscle tension which in turn acts like a giant spring squeezing together the bones of affected joints and placing even more pressure on surrounding nervous tissue. The result is more pain → more tension → more stress → more pain and you are locked into a vicious circle. There are many ways of relieving this type of muscular stress and breaking the tension barrier is often the first step on the road to recovery. We've seen already how manipulative treatment and massage can produce local relaxation, it's now time to consider ways of achieving long-term stress-busting which can, with a little practice, become a routine part of anyone's life-style and lead not only to speedier recovery, but also to long-term prevention of recurring back problems.

We all need to relax; not just by going on holiday once or twice a year, but by training ourselves consciously to relax for a short period each day. Relaxing does not mean just falling asleep: it is a conscious state in which all your muscles are relaxed one by one and your brain clears, to as close a state of emptiness as possible.

Some people relax actively, by going swimming, for example; others relax passively, by watching television. Watching television does not always secure the desired effect, however, since you achieve a state closer to sleep than relaxation, very often slumped in an uncomfortable posture or are overstimulated by the programmes.

What is relaxation?
When you are properly relaxed, a number of changes take place in your body. You will feel a sense of relaxed, sometimes heightened awareness, and a physical feeling of warmth and heaviness. Your heart rate will decrease (which is one of the reasons why true relaxation is good for you) and, because your heart is pumping blood more slowly, you will start to feel your entire body slowing down. Your blood sugar and blood fat levels, which increase in response to stress, will slowly return to a healthy level.

Relaxing for beginners
This simple exercise will slow your heart and breathing rate and help relax all those tense muscles which are causing you so much pain. You only need half an hour to begin with, and as you become practised, you'll need even less.

- Turn off the radio or television, disconnect the telephone and try to empty your mind of thought or emotion.

134

- In a warm room, lie flat on a very firm bed or on a rug on the floor. Close your eyes and take three deep, slow breaths in and out.
- Stretch your left leg along the floor away from your body as hard as you can, pointing your foot and contracting the calf, thigh, buttock and lower back muscles. Hold yourself in that position until you feel a slight trembling in the muscles, then relax. Repeat with the right leg; then with both legs, and relax.
- Stretch your left arm down your side, spreading your fingers and pushing from the big muscles at the back of the neck and shoulder, contracting all the muscles of the upper arm, forearm and hand. Relax.
- Repeat with the right arm and relax. Repeat with both arms and relax.
- Stretch both arms and legs together and relax.
- Take five deep breaths and repeat the cycle again. Repeat the cycle four more times.
- Relax totally for ten minutes, preferably with a blanket within reach, since body temperature may drop as a consequence of slower heart beat and lower breathing rates.

AUTOGENICS

This is a system of mental exercises, introduced in the 1930s by Dr. Johannes Schultz, German psychiatrist and neurologist, which is performed in order to relax the mind and body (autogenous means self-generating or originating within the body). Autogenic training (AT) is designed to switch off the stress 'fight or flight' response and switch on the rest, relaxation and recreation system associated with psychophysical relaxation. The exercises are extraordinarily simple and, once trained, you have a system which you can follow for life.

It is often recommended that you learn AT with a qualified practitioner, partly because a few people experience what is known as autogenic discharge, such as temporary twitching, feelings of dizziness, lethargy, anger, sadness or hilarity, which may be unexpected, although nothing to worry about.

The exercises
You will be taught to experience the sensations of heaviness and warmth, to regularise the heartbeat and the breathing, to induce a feeling of warmth in the abdomen and a feeling of coolness on the forehead. You will be instructed first to repeat, 'my right arm is heavy and warm, my heartbeat is calm and regular, my breathing even,' and so on, dealing first with the right arm and the five directions and so on through the body.

Autogenic training, when properly learned, produces a remarkable relief from tension and fatigue, both in day-to-day terms and in terms of eliminating stress that may have built up over years; this is thought to be the explanation for autogenic discharge. As with biofeedback, autogenics have been shown to be effective for any stress-related disorder, notably indigestion and ulcers, heart problems, asthma, migraine and anxiety.

BIOFEEDBACK

Biological feedback is essentially a system in which the body provides feedback or information about its condition by means of monitoring devices. The information you receive, which can be related to stress levels and anxiety, can be used to control and reduce these levels. The biofeedback instrument can measure skin temperature, muscle tone and even the amount of hydrochloric acid produced in the stomach.

The most common way in which the body provides feedback is through the sweat rate. Anxiety makes you sweat and sweat decreases the electrical resistance of the skin. This resistance can be measured through metal contacts or pads attached to the body and connected to a visual or audible signal, so that it is possible to tell when you are feeling stressed and anxious and, consequently, to make conscious efforts to control your body's stress levels.

Many people are not aware when they are under stress; indeed, one of the most pernicious aspects of stress is that you can become bound up in a situation and not recognise the damage you are doing to your body. The adrenalin builds up, without the facility for discharging itself either in fight or flight, and the body's heart rate, respiratory rate and levels of blood sugar and blood fats all increase to meet the challenge. All these changes contribute to heart disease.

The hardware
The different sorts of biofeedback machines include those that measure skin resistance (ESR), muscle tensions (EMG or electromyograph) and brain waves (EEG). Each of them will indicate, by buzzing at an increasingly high note as your stress level rises, what you will gradually be able to recognise for yourself without the aid of machinery: when you are calm, your skin is cool and dry (your skin resistance goes up) and the audible indicator will soften to a muffled click and then stop; when you are more agitated, the buzzing assumes a higher note; when you are really anxious, and your adrenalin is causing a cold sweat and palpitations, or when you are hot and flushed in response to the body's noradrenalin, which is released when you are angry, the buzzing becomes higher and higher until it screeches.

The biofeedback ideal is to learn to monitor your stress levels without gadgetry – when driving, for example – and to learn how to relax through deep breathing, good posture and observing regular daily relaxation periods. Biofeedback has become part of mainstream medicine and is used particularly in cardiac units and in migraine clinics. Its other applications include hypertension and insomnia.

MEDITATION

Meditation has always been an integral part of Indian religions, as well as Roman Catholicism (in saying the rosary), in Tibetan Buddhism (concentration upon the mandala) and in the Orthodox Church (concentration upon the icon). All forms of meditation seek to harmonise the way things are (reality) and the way they ought to be (the ideal). There is a great variety of systems of meditation and each put the emphasis to a greater or lesser degree on the main components, which are:

- to appreciate clearly the ideal order of things through greater awareness
- To develop receptiveness to that established order
- to be active in putting that order into practice.

In the West, the greatest emphasis has been placed on the vision of the ideal order, on visualising it in silent contemplation, and by concentrating upon it. All meditation techniques are based on the need to develop a particular kind of awareness, which can be described as a state of restful alertness where the mind is emptied of everything. To help the individual accomplish this, the various forms of meditation focus concentration onto a single subject and this concentration is accompanied by the continual repetition of a word or phrase, known as a mantra in some systems of meditation.

This rhythmic chanting is said to enhance meditation by exerting a vibrating and hypnotic effect upon the mind, leading to trance. Together with meditating itself, the trance is said to exert positive health effects, such as decreased heart rate and consequently lower blood pressure and a slower and more even respiratory rate, both of which will mitigate the possibility of heart disease, anxiety and stress-related disorders.

Types of meditation

Some forms of meditation are almost or totally devoid of content and the individual is encouraged to transcend thought entirely in order to cultivate a total receptiveness for the cosmic vision of the ideal order of things. These forms include the Japanese Zen Buddhism of 12th-century Chinese origin (which concentrates upon breathing, especially for beginners); the Taoist T'ai-Chi (which concentrates upon carefully designed and rhythmically precise movements to intensify and refine innate vital energy); and Transcendental Meditation (TM), a development of ancient Indian traditions, seeking to empty the mind entirely by entering the trance state, introduced to the West in 1959 by Maharishi Mahesh Yogi and enormously popular in the 1960s as a consequence of such luminaries as The Beatles taking it up.

Meditation for beginners

The following exercise is a synthesis of meditative systems devised by Dr. Herbert Benson of Harvard Medical School and has been found useful in treating stress.

- Sit, lie or recline in a comfortable position, making sure there are no external distractions such as radio or television.
- Shut your eyes.

- Relax all your muscles as in the basic relaxation exercise described earlier.
- Breathe deeply through your nose and try to clear your mind of all thought. Repeat the mantra word, 'one' either aloud or in your head. Breathe deeply and evenly and continue for 10–20 minutes, ignoring distracting thoughts and repeating the mantra.
- At the end, remain still, with your eyes shut for one or two minutes, then in the same position with your eyes open.

Some forms of meditation can cause sudden outbursts of emotion, such as tears and laughter. This is said to be a sign that the meditation is working.

YOGA

Yoga is used loosely in the West to describe many forms of relaxing exercise and meditation, accompanied by certain distinctive postures known as *asanas*. Yoga with a capital Y denotes the Hindu system of philosophy which aims at the mystical union of the self with the Supreme Being in a state of complete awareness and tranquillity through certain physical and mental exercises. Yoga can also mean, broadly, any method by which such awareness and tranquillity are attained, especially a course of related exercises and postures designed to promote a physical and spiritual well-being, but which is not necessarily formally religious.

The five main types of yoga, which are accepted by all schools of Indian philosophy are *karma yoga*, *jnana yoga*, *bhakti yoga*, *raja yoga* and *hatha yoga*. Hatha yoga is the basis of the modern practice of yoga in the West and is the system of yoga that concentrates upon longevity and health. There are other well-known types of yoga rest therapies that have become popular in the West, but these are merely the offshoots of hatha yoga that have been more energetically promoted and commercialised.

The Yoga system

Yoga is carried out in two levels: the first, known as *kriya yoga*, is the yoga of observances of physical accounts and this is carried out in five stages:

- adoption of restraint, or control, from evils (*yama*)
- adoption of religious observances (*niyama*)
- use of posture (*asana*) suitable for meditation
- restraint of breath or controlled breathing (*pranayama*)
- withdrawal of the senses from their objects (*pratya-hara*).

The second chief level of yoga, known as superior or royal yoga, is carried out in three stages:

- concentration (*dharana*) of the intelligence on an object
- meditation (*dhyana*) as an uninterrupted mental state and awareness of that object
- trance (*samadhi*) in which the individual is fully identified with the object of meditation, so that they become as one.

True Yoga, then, is a profoundly religious and spiritual system of philosophy which has existed in India for thousands of years and which has only comparatively recently been taken up in the West in an abridged form.

How can yoga help?

Many people take up yoga here simply because it teaches relaxation techniques, mobility and flexibility. The series of postures (*asanas*), which are an integral part of true Yoga, promote inner and outer harmony and grace and

141

have the added benefit of reducing stress and tension, making you sleep better and leaving you calm and relaxed with a clear, uncluttered mind.

Yoga is suitable for people of all ages from young children to the elderly and arthritic. It is a particularly good form of exercise for the elderly because it is fairly gentle. It should be done regularly for maximum benefit and, when starting out it is better to have personal supervision from a teacher before practising at home.

Set aside 15–20 minutes each day for deep breathing and some of the simple *asanas* Many people have found that these basic exercises have helped them to cope better with daily pressures and the relief of tension, without even moving on to more advanced postures.

Whatever the origins of yoga and its various systems, and indeed of meditation as well, there can be no doubt that these therapies are not only benign – provided that they do not relieve the participants of too much in fees – but can be positively health-giving in their role of reducing stress. For the many people who suffer from chronic stress symptoms, such as back pain, migraine, asthma and hypertension, hobbies, exercise and beneficial sleep are not enough. For them the answer lies in systematic relaxation. Some of the simple techniques of relaxation are useful for almost everyone, however, since temporary stress, at least, is sometimes unavoidable.

HYPNOTHERAPY

Many of us talk and act as if our conscious mind were the most important part of us, running everything in our mind and body, making decisions and permitting us to do things. In contrast, the unconscious mind is often regarded as something fairly peripheral, doing rather vague things of which we are not really aware. A moment's thought begins to make it clear that the opposite is true; the unconscious mind is constantly working, monitoring all the physical and psychological functions of the mind and the body, from blood pressure and hormone levels to states of hunger and fatigue, even when we are asleep. The conscious mind, on the other hand, only deals with the 'here and now', and indeed turns off when we are asleep.

The unconscious mind also copes with much of our memory of what has happened, remembering a very large proportion of our experiences – far more than we could ever consciously remember. Hypnosis is a method whereby the practitioner can speak to the unconscious mind directly, and can therefore communicate with that part of the mind that controls everything from perception to memory. It is, essentially, a complex process of attentive, retentive *concentration* with diminished awareness of surroundings.

Hypnosis is not really normal sleep: it is better to regard it as 'turning down the volume' of the conscious mind, so as to be able to gain direct access to the unconscious mind. With this sort of direct access, 'reality testing' is disconnected, and the distinction between the imaginary and the real disappears, so that the mind reacts to the imaginary (in other words, whatever is suggested to it) as if it were real. It can therefore be an extremely valuable tool in a programme of treatment, but it cannot be regarded as an end in itself.

How hypnotherapy works

Imagery produces responses in us in everyday life, and can affect our behaviour: and this is what the hypnosis practitioner uses, while making the imagery more powerful, more specific and more 'real' to the person being hypnotised. Adequate preparation is important, and the practitioner will spend some time discussing the problem that has driven the patient to seek help. He or she will then explain what will happen in hypnosis and take the patient into the first trance.

In the first stage of the trance, a rapport is established, with the patient becoming receptive to the practitioner's signals, such as concentrating upon an object or upon a spot on the ceiling, for example, to enter the full trance. (This sort of visual fixation tires the eyes and the conscious mind very quickly.) The practitioner indicates the likely mental and physical phenomena, such as drowsiness, that will be experienced. Provided that the patient is receptive, he or she starts to experience the mind and body effects predicted by the practitioner. The next stage of trance can be called the plunge, in which the patient more or less relinquishes their critical faculties and gives themself up to the practitioner.

Once in a trance, then things may be suggested to the patient that his conscious mind will remember. He can be taught quicker methods of going into a trance, so it is much easier in future sessions, and the level of trance can be made progressively deeper.

The patient may experience sensory changes such as parasthesia (the sensation of pins and needles), analgesia, anaesthesia, partial amnesia and, after the treatment is over, compliance with simple signals that the practitioner will have arranged during the period of hypnosis, while the connection between reality and imagery is broken.

The advantages of hypnosis
The value of hypnotherapy lies in its ability to cut through the patient's verbal evasions or discussion, in which it could take hours to resolve a single issue, as it penetrates the unconscious and releases information which might otherwise be withheld.

The true hypnotherapist will not promote the instant cure – the stage hypnotist's domain – as they work usually over four to five sessions by altering ingrained patterns of thought and behaviour. A compulsive eater, therefore, is treated so that he or she not only eats less but deals with the fundamental issues that gave rise to the overeating in the first place.

It is important that the therapist takes time with the patient, with the goal of altering these deeply ingrained patterns of thought: the smoker who enjoys smoking but who is addicted to the nicotine and would prefer to give up may be treated successfully and quickly. The smoker who uses the habit as an outlet for some deep-seated anxiety will probably need longer to deal not only with the habit itself but to confront the psychological component of the problem. If that problem is not dealt with, the patient could inadvertently discover a different outlet.

It has already been said that the unconscious remembers a great deal of our experiences – possibly everything. Under hypnosis we can find these memories, learning about experiences that have affected us in the past, and working through memories which may be repressed but which may yet still give us pain.

Lastly, hypnosis is a very pleasant experience; and it will teach you things about relaxation and coping with the world which will almost certainly be of a wider application than the problem that originally made you seek treatment.

HEALING HERBS

If you think that herbal remedies are just old wives' tales, you may be surprised to know that 25 per cent of all prescriptions written by doctors are for medicines wholly or partially derived from plants. These range from the most powerful pain-killers like morphine to simple indigestion mixtures containing peppermint oil. There are many herbal medicines which are effective in the relief of back pain and these are generally those which have an anti-inflammatory effect: plants like the humble dandelion, willow, primula, and the more exotic African Devil's Claw.

For the relief of rheumatism and arthritis the most effective herbal remedy is **BioStrath Willow Formula**, a combination of willow and primula. The Belgian product **Harpago** is a liquid extract of Devil's Claw used for centuries by the bushmen of the Namibian Kalahari Desert to relieve aches and pains. **Meadowsweet** contains the same chemical as aspirin and an infusion of its flowers makes an excellent tea for the same purpose. **Ginger tea** is made by grating an inch of fresh root into a mug of boiling water, leave it to stand for ten minutes, strain it and then add a little honey. Drink a cup each morning as this has a dramatic effect on the circulation and will speed the healing process of damaged tissues in the back.

A poultice of **hot cabbage leaves** applied to the painful area has been a traditional European treatment for arthritis and rheumatism for centuries and remains an effective treatment. Essential oils of **lavender**, **pine** or **juniper** can be added to a hot bath – maximum ten drops – for their relaxing and circulatory effect and five drops of any one added to 50ml of sunflower seed oil is an effective mixture for massaging into painful joints and muscles.

One of the most effective natural anti-inflammatories is **Evening Primrose Oil** and, when combined with fish oil, as it is in Efamol Marine, it can be a great help in the treatment of arthritically induced backache. It's interesting that neither the Eskimos nor the coastal New Zealand Maoris appear to suffer from arthritis. The Eskimos' traditional food is whale blubber and that of the Maoris is the New Zealand green-lipped mussel. There are now commercially available extracts of these mussels, Seatone, and many varieties of fish oil on the market.

146

Eating oily fish is always good for people with arthritic joints whose diet should also include fresh fruit, almonds, potatoes, millet, cabbage, carrots and, contrary to popular opinion, strawberries, raspberries and cherries. One of the most valuable and freely available plants for the treatment of arthritis is the **stinging nettle**. Gather the young plants – away from the roadside or dogs to avoid contamination – wearing gloves, and make them into soup like any other vegetable, or use them to make nettle tea by chopping a handful of leaves, add a cup of boiling water and leave to stand for at least ten minutes before straining and drinking.

All arthritics should avoid red meat, red wine, sherry, port, Madeira, and large amounts of refined sugars and carbohydrates. Anyone suffering from rheumatoid arthritis should also avoid dairy products for a few weeks as this can make a dramatic difference in some patients. If it doesn't help, put them back in the diet. If it does help, then get some professional advice about replacing the calcium which you will be missing out on by avoiding these normally excellent food sources.

CHAPTER 10

Practical Things that Help

Back pain can be caused by several things which you would never think could be so damaging to your health. These things are so normal we take them for granted, never imagining that they could be harming our backs by misuse. These things are your car, your bed, your sofa, your TV set and, last but by no means least, your feet.

IS YOUR CAR A PAIN IN THE BACK?

Whether you are a professional driver or a weekend pleasure seeker, eight hours behind the wheel can damage your spine. A while ago, I enjoyed a round trip up and down the M1 from London to Ilkeston in Derbyshire. On the way back I paused for a little light refreshment, and more importantly, a break from the monotony of the motorway. Taking a short stroll round the Watford Gap car park to restore some circulation to the legs I was surprised by the number of drivers of all ages, shapes, sizes and both sexes, who eased themselves out of their cars, hauled themselves upright on the door frame, grimaced and rubbed the small of their backs.

Backache, it seems, is an occupational hazard for drivers. I don't know why I was so surprised, I see dozens of patients each month whose back pain is caused by car seats, so I should have expected the motorway car park to look like an osteopath's waiting room!

A recent survey of 675 patients attending osteopaths for back pain revealed that 84 per cent of them related their problem to driving. Half of them said that within an hour's driving they were uncomfortable and 95 per cent of them had pain and discomfort after sitting behind the wheel for three hours. Only 25 per cent of automatic drivers suffered backache compared with 70 per cent who drove manuals, so the first improvement you could make is to switch to an automatic car as soon as you can.

When choosing a car watch out for pedals or steering wheel which are offset – sit in the seat and see if you have to move your legs and arms to the left rather than having them pointing straight ahead when you're in the driving position. Also make sure that the seat has adequate lumbar and side support and that you can adjust it to suit your height and size.

A regular programme of back exercises to keep your spine mobile and the muscles in good shape, will make a big difference. On long journeys make sure that you stop for five minutes every hour, get out of the car and have a good stretch and walk about.

Most people choose their car for all the wrong reasons. Apart from price and running costs, what did you consider first – colour, top speed, performance, extras, resale value? All wrong. First, look at the driving seat which you're going to be in throughout the life of your car. Uncomfortable seats cause fatigue as well as pain, and fatigue causes accidents. The more comfortable you are, the better you are going to drive, so how do you choose the best seat for you? Not in the car showroom, or on a ten-minute whizz around the block, with an enthusiastic salesman sitting beside you. You must drive the car for at least an hour, make sure that you can reach all the controls easily, that the angle of the pedals suits you, that the seat can be adjusted so that your driving position is just as you like it, that the head restraints have enough movement to fit your height and body shape.

The seat must move easily, without breaking your finger nails, the squab (the bit you put your bottom on) should not be too long or short for your thighs, and ideally should be adjustable so you can alter the angle. Lateral support is vital, each time you go round a corner, the body tenses to keep you in your seat. This repeated strain can be the trigger of muscle spasm, and lead to pain as well as stress.

Pay special attention to the head restraint. I see so many drivers using these as neck rests – the perfect way to guarantee a whiplash injury at best, a broken neck at worst. The point of contact must be level with the ears, and the distance between the back of your skull and the rest ought to be no more than two or three inches. The whole restraint needs enough adjustment for your comfort and safety, both up and down, and forwards and backwards. In the perfect position, your head is supported at all times, which avoids a lot of the strain on the neck muscles and the resulting pain and headaches.

As an osteopath I was delighted to hear of the Government's plans for a dramatic increase in the number of motorway service stations throughout the country. It's a great pity that we have not adopted the European idea of having rest areas on our motorway system too. If you drive in Switzerland you'll find many of these with toilet facilities, picnic areas and best of all, simple exercise equipment complete with instructions to help the driver eliminate fatigue, get the circulation going again and limber up those stiff and aching joints and muscles. There's no doubt in my mind that the capital cost involved would be more than offset by the reduction in accidents and a sharp fall in the numbers of drivers and their passengers needing medical attention and time off work as a result of back pain.

Osteopaths throughout the UK are growing more and more concerned about the ever-growing incidence of back pain which is inseparably linked to driving. The survey quoted above was conducted by giving questionnaires to 675 patients in osteopath's surgeries right across the country. These were completed over a three-week period spanning August and September 1993 and, apart from the figures already mentioned, around 75 per cent of the drivers who suffered discomfort were complaining of low back pain and 20 per cent reported symptoms in the legs or feet.

One osteopath, Bryan McIlwraith, has made a detailed study of the way in which the design of the modern motor car has developed. He believes that changes in car construction have a negative effect on the driver's posture which in turn causes muscular strain and back pain. The root of the problems started with the Mini in 1959. Because of its small size, exceptional manoeuvrability, revolutionary road-holding and general handling – those of us old enough to remember the excitement of driving the first Minis can testify to that – the Mini's designer Sir Alec Issigonis made a number of compromises that were to influence car design for the next 30 years. The front wheels were moved closer to the driver occupying space in the foot well where the pedals were traditionally mounted.

Sir Alec's way of solving this problem was to shift the pedals closer to the centre of the car, but this also moved them slightly to the side of the driver. This now commonplace pedal offset is the acceptable standard for small car design. For this reason the driver's position has been altered so that the right leg remains slightly twisted and deviated from the hip joint, thereby placing strain on the lower region of the back in order to keep the foot on the accelerator pedal.

McIlwraith's studies also show that many modern cars

have steering wheels offset as well and he maintains that there is no justification for this whatsoever. The wheel in some cars is not directly in front of the driver but can be offset to the left by as much as 5cm which means that the entire shoulder girdle rotates slightly to the left as you hold the wheel in both hands. This creates stresses in the upper part of the back as well.

Another concern which appeared in the study was the lack of headroom in many modern cars. As Brian points out: 'In pursuit of a streamlined shape to enhance fuel economy the designers have lowered the roof line of the modern car which means that the taller driver must be placed even lower in the bucket seat'. To compensate for this limited headroom, taller drivers are forced to slouch down into the seat which increases the likelihood of back and thigh pain.

For some drivers any one of these design factors can cause a problem, and all of them together would probably produce pain and discomfort in the fittest, healthiest, most mobile driver imaginable. It's not easy for the untrained eye to spot these specific features and in the excitement of acquiring your new pride and joy, it's all too easy to ignore a seemingly minor discomfort because you've already persuaded yourself that this is the particular car you are longing to park outside your front door. Brian McIlwraith has devised four simple tests which should be performed before you part with your hard-earned cash.

1. The Praying Test
Sit in the driver's seat and put your palms together in front of you with fingers pointing forwards. If the steering wheel is not offset then the tips of your fingers will be pointing towards the centre of the wheel. The offset steering wheel encourages rotation of the middle part of the spine and leads to muscle and joint strain.

2. The Fist Test

Adjust the driving seat to your most comfortable position for normal driving. Make sure you can reach the brake pedal and depress the clutch without stretching if the car is not automatic. Now make a fist with your left hand keeping your thumb on the outside of the index finger and put your fist on top of your head. If there is not enough room between your head and the car roof and you can only squeeze your flat hand between the two, then there is probably not enough headroom. This tends to make the driver slouch in the seat putting excessive strain on the spine and thighs.

3. The Look Down Test

Place both hands on the steering wheel in the '10 to 2' position and look down at your legs. If the steering wheel is centrally located you will see equal amounts of each leg. If, however, the steering wheel is offset to the left, you will see more of the left thigh but part of the right leg will be obscured by the right arm showing that the whole shoulder girdle is rotated to the right.

4. The Right Leg Test

You should do this test after you've been driving for 10 to 15 minutes. Stop the car, look down and study the position of your right leg. Is it raised above the level of the left one, or has it fallen outwards to the edge of the seat? Is your right foot in line with the thigh as it should be in the perfect driving position, or has it inched across more towards the centre of the car? Any irregularity in the position of the foot or leg can lead to strain of the leg muscles, the knee joint, the hip joint, the sacroiliac joint and general stress on the lower spine.

If the car you want passes these simple tests then it's reasonable to assume that it is a suitable car for you. If you make sure that you always use these tests when buying a new car your risk of driver's backache will be greatly reduced. If you're sharing the car with your spouse, partner or teenage offspring, you have an additional set of problems. I would suggest that the car should be ideal for the person who's going to spend most time driving it, then at least one of you will be OK. If you try to compromise, you end up giving everybody a pain in the back.

If you are stuck with a seat that gives you a pain in the back, don't scrap the car as there are things you can do to improve your back and the seat. Maybe you can't afford to fit a Recaro – the best of all the seats on the market, from £500 to £1000 – but you can turn to Putnams (see address in reference section), who made their name by installing special seats in London's black cabs. They produce a range of inexpensive and anatomically sound supports. Their Superest will fill in the hollow at the base of the spine, and provide a firm lateral grip to combat the G forces of cornering. The cost, less than ten gallons, is around £23.

The Bakrest is contoured foam on a solid base, and can be moved up and down on the back of your seat so that the support is where you need it most, and all for around £18. If your seat has seen better days, and dips and sags before you even put your backside on it, then you need a Putnams Seat Topper. Designed to fill in the empty spaces and improve your posture in a worn seat, it is yours for around £18.

If you're off to buy a new car this weekend, then my advice is take an osteopath with you. If you can't manage that, then at least take this book with you and read it again while you sit in the driving seat.

YOU MAKE THE BED, YOU LIE IN IT

When did you last look at your bed? I mean – have a really

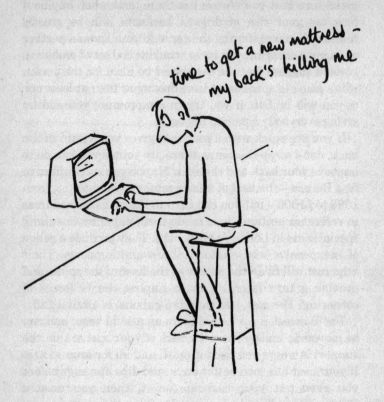

time to get a new mattress – my back's killing me

close look at your bed. Over a 20-year period you might have had 3 washing machines, 2 fridges, 4 vacuum cleaners, 5 different cars, but many couples will still be sleeping in the same bed they had the day they got married. A bed that sags in the middle, that rolls you into one another and does not support your spine. Don't be taken in by all those advertisements for magical 'orthopaedic' beds that are very expensive and recommended by experts. All the leading bed manufacturers make excellent extra-firm beds for those with back problems. Take your time, try them out and don't be hassled by sales reps knocking on your door and don't be embarrassed about lying on the bed in your local furniture store for a good half an hour in different positions. After all, you are going to spend a third of your life for the next twenty years in it.

Even turning the mattress can make a pretty dramatic difference and if there is a significant weight gap between you and your partner, make sure you turn it side to side as well as top to bottom. If you do it properly the top left-hand corner upper surface ends up as the bottom right-hand corner lower surface. If you already have a back problem, don't do this little chore yourself, ideally, find a couple of strong lads to do it for you.

The sort of bed you choose will depend on your own personal preferences, but the ideal is a very firm base with a good quality, firm mattress which should have a soft yielding surface. Few people are comfortable sleeping on a mattress which is as hard as a board, and just as few will enjoy sinking into an old-fashioned, three-foot-thick mattress with the consistency of blancmange. Good quality foam is excellent – a six-foot block of cheap upholstery polystyrene on a few reclaimed wooden pallets is not. Good mattresses on slatted wooden bases which have a slight spring are increasingly popular and excellent and the current vogue for the Japanese futon is another good alternative for healthy sleep. These very low beds however create their own problems when it comes to making them – see below.

Of course, it is still possible to go to one of the great English furniture makers like Heals in London and have your bed made to your own specification, complete with horsehair-stuffed mattress, that's assuming you've got several thousand pounds to spare. One exciting new development in beds has grown out of the American space programme. A specially developed visco-elastic foam was created to solve problems with the astronauts' couches. These had to be supportive enough to sustain enormous

G-force pressures at take-off, yet at the same time be soft and resilient for many hours in the same position. Now a Swedish company has developed the original material and is marketing the Tempur mattress with great success. The unique properties of this foam avoid the discomfort of hard mattresses and the spinal stresses of sagging ones. The mattress responds to the combination of bodyweight and warmth, moulding itself around the contours of the body giving overall support and minimum pressure. When you get up the mattress returns to its normal shape. I haven't yet tried one for myself but I have seen the material and some patients have already reported great benefits from using this type of mattress.

Even if you avoid backache by sleeping in a good bed, you can get it by making it. Very low beds pose extra problems, as do bunk beds, beds in corners and fold-away beds which are a strain to move. Never stretch across the bed to tuck in the other side. Never bend at the waist, lift the mattress and stretch forward to tuck the sheets underneath. Never stand on the stepladder and stretch into the farthest corner of the top bunk, or crouch bent double to reach the other side of the bottom bunk. If you're tucking in sheets and blankets, kneel on one knee so that the underside of the mattress is at waist height. Pull the bed away from the wall – all beds should be on castors – to avoid the straight-backed bending across it.

Many of the problems associated with bedmaking can be avoided by using fitted sheets on the bottom and duvets on the top, though the problems of getting the duvet into the duvet cover whilst not being harmful to the back can be very fraying to the nerves (see page 104). It's worth considering a higher bed if you already have a back problem or if you are getting on in years, as they are easier to get in and out of and a lot easier to make.

One doesn't hear too much about water beds these days, but for those of you who feel tempted, I've never thought of them as particularly good for people with back problems. Whilst they can provide some quite interesting sensations they can also be the cause of very disturbed sleep if your partner is restless, even more so if your partner is heavier than you as well as restless. What's more, they tend to provide a very rigid surface contact almost as bad as an overinflated lilo. Their enormous weight sometimes means reinforcing the bedroom floor, so all in all, not a great idea.

Pillows are a bedroom item which frequently get ignored, usually to the detriment of your neck and shoulders. For those suffering from severe neck problems as a result of injury or arthritis, the special neck pillows can be a great boon, but in general the ideal pillow is the best quality feather pillow that you can afford. Sadly for those of you with allergies, you are likely to be limited to foam pillows on which your head bounces up and down like a cork in water. My advice is to try a feather pillow covered in one of the new materials like Intervent (from Boots) which allows moisture to pass through but not the droppings of the house dust mite which are the cause of most domestic allergic reactions.

One or at most two good quality feather pillows can be moulded exactly into the shape of your neck and shoulder, keeping your spine nice and level no matter which position you choose to sleep in.

You do spend a third of your life in bed. Bed is restorative, comforting, healing and it can also be fun. A new bed is a long-term investment and just because it isn't 'on show' to most visitors to your home, don't skimp. Buy the best quality you can afford and you'll go a long way to saving oodles of money by looking after your back, not being off work with a backache and not having to visit your local osteopath.

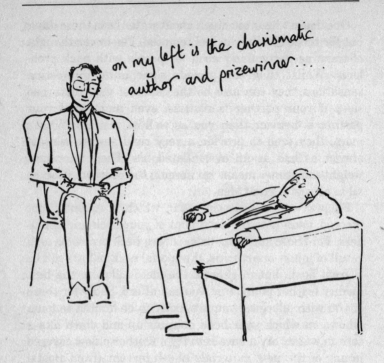

on my left is the charismatic author and prizewinner....

SOFA, SO GOOD?

Soft armchairs with low backs and no support are one of the worst enemies of the spine. When you fall asleep the head lolls down and to one side and as the shoulders slump, the lower part of the spine curves over like a sack of potatoes tied in the middle. Modern furniture designers have a great deal to answer for. Earlier craftsmen had a much better sense of what suited the human anatomy and the Queen Anne style high-backed wing armchair was designed to support the back and the head in great comfort. The same is true of dining chairs and sofas. Ultramodern designs often slope down from front to back leaving you to stretch forward to the dining table, whilst the sofas make you perch on the edge in great discomfort or tip back with your feet in the air and your shoulders, neck and head lolling behind you over a back support that barely reaches your waist.

Fashions in furniture come and go, but the comfort and good design of traditional English style has never gone out of fashion. If you insist on being à la mode, do at least sit in the furniture you're going to buy for long enough to make sure that it suits your own body structure. Buying two or three identical armchairs is nearly always a disaster as few couples are identical shapes or sizes. His and hers is the best solution.

FRED'S STORY

Fred was 46 when I first saw him as a patient. He had a sedentary job, he took no exercise, was a little overweight and suffered from mild but nagging backache. The reason he consulted me was not because of his back which he said he could live with, and had done so for the past three or four years, but because of the recent onset of pain and stiffness in his neck. After several treatments he reported that the pain was certainly better for the rest of the day after his visit, but by the time he went to bed the same night it had all come back. Detailed questioning about his life-style, his habits, and an almost minute by minute analysis of his whole day failed to reveal anything which could be the trigger of this pain. X-rays showed no injury or arthritis and both of us were getting more than a little frustrated by his lack of progress.

It must have been Fred's fifth or sixth visit when he came with his wife who asked if she could watch him having his treatment. While I was working on Fred's neck and shoulder muscles I was explaining to Mrs Fred how strange it was that we hadn't been able to identify the cause of his problem. She leapt to her feet and shouted at her unfortunate spouse, at that moment lying face down on my couch, 'Does this mean that you haven't told him about the armchair?' Silence from Fred, as the blush spread to the tips of his ears. The explanation was simple but he was too embarrassed to admit it. Every night Fred came home from work, had a couple of whiskies and soda, ate his meal, sat in his favourite armchair to watch the *News at Ten*, and woke up at around three in the morning. His wife had long since given up trying to get him to bed at a sensible time and she knew that sleeping for hours cradled in the embrace of his 20-year-old, overstuffed and very soft chair was almost certainly the cause of the problem.

I am pleased to report that Fred's old chair went on the bonfire and although he still falls asleep in front of the telly, both his back and neck are hugely better as he enjoys the support of a modern reproduction of the wing armchair.

WHERE DO YOU PUT YOUR TV?

Let's assume that you've been out and bought yourself a really smashing high-backed armchair which supports the whole of your spine and enables you to sit with your head resting on the back of the chair in a totally relaxed and comfortable position. Imagine yourself sitting in the chair with your head supported and staring straight at the wall. The spot which you're looking at will be somewhere between four and five feet off the ground, depending on your height and the height of the chair.

Now look at the centre of your TV screen. Almost certainly that is two feet six inches, or at the most three feet, above the ground. In order to watch your favourite programme you need to bend your head forwards and downwards, stretching the muscles at the back of the neck and shoulders and flexing the joints in the upper part of your spine. A few hours in this position, especially when you do it most nights of the week, establish abnormal patterns of muscle tension which lead to headaches, neckaches, pain in the shoulder muscles and upper part of the back and can even be the trigger for migraine attacks.

Why everyone puts their TV in such a ridiculous position is beyond me. Just to make matters worse, the video machine is under the TV and these days is often joined by the control boxes for the satellite dish. So, not content with straining your neck watching the wretched thing, viewers then spend time grovelling on the floor trying to struggle with the intricacies of setting the timer, changing the tapes or resetting the clock every time there's a power cut. If you've already got backache, all this is guaranteed to make you feel even worse. If you've had it in the past it's a pretty good way to make sure you get it again in the future, and if you haven't had it yet it's bound to increase your chances of becoming yet another statistic in the tables of back sufferers.

Your television set should be placed on a higher shelf with the video and satellite bits and pieces next to it. Make sure you put the video tapes at the same height so that you can sort through them in a comfortable position, avoiding yet further back strain. By the way, another good reason for raising up your electronic equipment from floor level is that it protects them from dog and cat hairs, dust and dirt – all of which do nothing to improve their performance. If you think none of this applies to you because you've got a remote control set or three, remember that it won't change the tapes, its batteries have probably run out and you don't understand which button to push anyway. American research has shown that from the day you acquire a remote control for your TV you will gain two pounds in weight each year just because you're not getting up and down from your armchair to change the channels.

Most homes now have at least two if not three TVs and many of these end up in the bedroom. Bedroom telly watching is another back disaster unless you do it right. Propping yourself up on eight pillows, watching the small screen perched on the dressing-table stool, and peering over humps in the duvet created by your partner is a sure way of putting excessive strain on the lower lumbar region of your spine. The ideal bedroom telly is wall-mounted on the sort of bracket which is adjustable in every direction. You can watch it lying comfortably on your back with no strain whatsoever. If you are suffering an enforced period of bedrest due to a bad back anyway, it helps to while away the hours of boredom. This is one situation in which the remote control set is indispensable. It avoids all the arguments about who's going to get up and turn the thing off, or being woken at three in the morning by the glaring white screen and the hideous hiss and crackle.

The television is a major factor in the relentless rise of back pain. It chains millions of people to their armchairs (see above), it encourages children to be physically

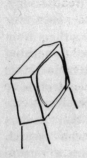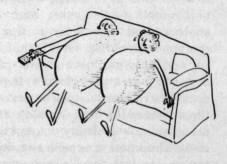

inactive and leaving aside all questions of taste, programme quality and psychological effects, it has a devastating impact on the amount of physical activity that we pursue as a nation. The human frame is designed for movement, not inertia and in terms of general mobility it's an absolute truism to say 'use it or lose it'.

HAP-HAP-HAP-HAP-HAP-HAP-HAPPY FEET

Comfortable and healthy feet are a vital cornerstone in the healthy backpack. They're the only ones you'll get, so take care of them. Comfortable shoes and attention to hygiene are the best ways of ensuring healthy feet. Uncomfortable poorly fitting shoes will cause foot problems like bunions and corns, and will also adversely affect your posture, creating fatigue, discomfort and even pain.

Do not wear high heels as a matter of habit as they tip your weight forward. This exaggerates the inward curve at the base of your spine – the lumbar lordosis – and also leads to compression of the toes as your weight is thrown down into the front of the shoe. Furthermore, constant wearing of high heels can make the muscles and tendons at the back of the ankle shorten. This reduces free movement of the ankle joint and can also affect your posture and walking.

Cheap trainers made entirely of synthetic material and with inadequate internal supporting structures are a disaster. They don't fit properly, they don't prop up the arches of the foot, and they cause excessive sweating. Good quality trainers are expensive but can be a boon. The latest air-cushioned designs absorb impact, protect the feet and also the spine and intervertebral discs. They can be wonderful for back sufferers, the only problem is persuading older members of the community that it's OK to wear 'gym shoes' when you go out to do the shopping. I tell them that their grandchildren will think they're very with-it.

Look after your feet by washing them at least once a day with warm water and a mild but not medicated perfumed soap. Dry carefully between the toes to avoid athlete's foot, which can also be painful and cause postural changes. If you have the common problem of sweaty feet, wash them morning and evening and use a very light sprinkle of foot powder. Remove rough skin with a smooth pumice stone and if you have a lot of dry skin on your feet rub in a little lanolin-based cream night and morning. Keep your toenails short, cutting them straight across with proper nail clippers not scissors and don't snip down the sides of the nail which is likely to cause infection and ingrowing toenails. Keep your clippers clean by wiping with disinfectant and drying well after use, and make sure you wipe them with a little disinfectant before using them next time.

If you wear proper shoes and look after your feet carefully, you shouldn't be bothered by corns or bunions. Regular visits to a State Registered chiropodist are an excellent idea and at the first sign of any foot problems, that's the person you should consult immediately.

FREDA'S STORY

Freda Jones was 76 when her daughter first brought her to my surgery. She was a bubbling, energetic, cheerful pensioner leading a totally independent life and enjoying gardening, cooking and the occasional game of bowls at her village club. That was, until the backache struck. For seven months she had endured chronic pain at the bottom of her spine which spread through her left buttock and into her left leg as far down as her foot. When she lay down in bed or sat on a rigid kitchen chair she was fairly comfortable, but as soon as she tried to be active the pain started. Poor Freda had been through the entire medical mill and after the usual bedrest, pain-killers, physio, stronger pain-killers, X-rays and finally a battery of tests for all sorts of terrible diseases they couldn't find anything.

In the end poor Freda was sent home to live with her backache and to face the prospect of life without all her favourite pastimes. She became dependent on her daughter and home helps, very depressed and was left wondering whether life was really worth living.

It had been a real struggle for Freda's daughter to get her to see me, as understandably she had quite enough of being poked and prodded without anyone coming up with a solution to her problem. We had a long talk about the way in which her problem had changed her life and then got down to the examination. After looking at Freda's posture and a thorough study of her spine I looked at her shoes. The heel of the left shoe was worn down twice as much as the one on the right and I asked whether this had always happened to her shoes. 'Oh no,' she replied, 'only since I had the corn on the other foot.' And, sure enough, in the centre of the ball of her right foot was a large inflamed corn. Freda used to get regular visits from a chiropodist, but her local health service were no longer able to supply this service and the poor woman had suffered for months. The pain made her limp, the limp affected her posture, and the change in posture set up a whole pattern of muscular strains which caused her pain.

The happy outcome was that Freda's daughter took her to a chiropodist to have the corn removed and within a month she was back to normal, enjoying the garden and her bowls. I relate this story not because I want you to think how clever I am – I'm certainly not – but to illustrate the importance of the osteopath's holistic approach to the patient. Freda had never thought to mention her corn and no one else had ever looked at her feet.

Barefoot exercises
Happy feet can be maintained by doing these simple barefoot exercises.

1. Practise picking up pencils with your toes – you can do it while you're reading, relaxing or even watching TV.
2. Straighten your legs in front of you and loop a wide elastic band across both big toes. Starting with your feet together gradually turn them outwards keeping the heels in contact till your feet are in the '10 to 2' position. This stretches the elastic band and straightens the big toes, exercising the joint and reducing the risk of bunions. Repeat the movement twenty-five times.
3. Using an old-fashioned wooden rolling pin, put it on the floor at right angles to your foot. Stand behind an upright chair supporting your weight with your hands on the back of it. Put the toes of one foot on the rolling pin keeping your heel on the floor. Then roll your foot across the rolling pin so that your toes are on the floor and your heel is on the top of it. Roll backwards and forwards fifteen times, pressing down quite firmly to stretch the long arch of the foot. Then turn the rolling pin parallel to the foot and put the whole foot on top of it, rolling from side to side gripping with the toes. This exercises the lateral muscles and the ankle joint. Do this fifteen times, then repeat both exercises with the other foot.

This simple programme of foot care is just as vital

whether you are a sedentary office worker, a nurse walking the wards all day, a postman, travelling salesman or soldier. The heavy foot user will benefit just as much as the couch potato. Foot care is essential to back care.

Useful Addresses

For information about acupuncture, chiropractic, home-
opathy, medical herbalism, naturopathy and osteopathy
contact:

The Council for Complementary and Alternative Medicine (CCAM),
179 Gloucester Place,
London NW1 6DX
(071 724 9103)

British College of Naturopathy and Osteopathy,
6 Netherhall Gardens,
London NW3 5RR
(071 435 6464)
(For outpatient clinic at very reduced rates and the only
full-time degree course combining naturopathy and osteopathy)

The General Council and Register of Naturopaths,
6 Netherhall Gardens,
London NW3 5RR
(071 435 6464)

The British Acupuncture Association,
34 Alderney Street,
London SW1V 4EV
(071 834 1012)

The Society of Teachers of the Alexander Technique,
Suite 20,
10 London House,
266 Fulham Road,
London SW10 9EL
(071 351 0828)

The British Chiropractic Association,
29 Whitley Street
Reading,
Berks RG2 0EG
(0734 757557)

National Institute of Medical Herbalists,
9 Palace Gate,
Exeter,
Devon EX1 1JA
(0392 426022)

The General Council and Register of Osteopaths,
56 London Road,
Reading,
Berkshire RG1 4SQ
(0734 576585)

The Disabled Living Foundation,
380 Harrow Road,
London W9 2HU
(071 289 6911)

The British League Against Rheumatism
3 St. Andrews Place,
Regents Park,
London NW1 4LB
(071 224 3739)
An umbrella group for Arthritis Care, the Scoliosis

Association, and the National Ankylosing Spondylitis
Society

National Back Pain Association,
31–33 Park Road,
Teddington,
Middx TW11 0AB
(081 977 5474)

SUPPLIERS

Putnam's,
Eastern Wood Road,
Langage Industrial Estate,
Plymptom,
Devon PL7 5ET
(0752 345678)

Tempur-Pedic (UK) Ltd.,
Monomark House,
27 Old Gloucester Street,
London WC1N 3XX
(071 867 8436)

The Back Store,
330 King Street,
Hammersmith,
London W6 0RR
(071 741 5022)

The Royal Horticultural Society,
80 Vincent Square,
London SW1P 2PE
(071 834 4333)
For advice on disabled gardening

Keep Able,
Fleming Close,
Park Farm,
Wellingborough,
Northants NN8 6UF
Head offices for catalogue of every practical aid you can
think of

The Society for Horticultural Therapy,
Trunkwell Park,
Beech Hill,
Reading RG7 2AT
(0734 884844)
Special tools and equipment together with useful advice

The Council on Chiropractic Education (CCE),
4401 Westown Parkway,
Suite 120,
West Des Moines,
Iowa 50266,
U.S.A.
(010 1 515 226 9001)

The American Osteopathic Association,
142 East Ohio Street,
Chicago,
Illinois IL60611,
U.S.A.
(010 1 312 280 5800)

The American Academy of Osteopathy,
3500 DePauw Boulevard,
Suite 1080,
Indianapolis IN 46268-139,
U.S.A.
(010 1 317 879 1881)

Canadian Memorial Chiropractic College,
1900 Bayview Ave,
Toronto,
Ontario,
Canada M4G 3E6
(010 1 416 482-2340)

Macquarie University,
Centre for Chiropractic and Osteopathy,
P.O. Box 178,
Summerhill,
New South Wales,
Australia 2130
(011-61-2-798-7952)

Royal Melbourne Institute of Technology,
School of Chiropractic and Osteopathy,
Plenty Road,
Bundoora,
Victoria,
Australia 3083
(011-61-3-468-2440)

Australian Osteopathic Association,
Federal Office,
1/267 Castlereagh Street,
Sydney,
New South Wales 2000,
Australia
(010 612 264 9171)

Index

Sexual Awareness

Enhancing Sexual Pleasure

Barry and Emily McCarthy

ILLUSTRATED   NEW UNEXPURGATED EDITION

This book is written to show individuals and couples how to enhance their sexual pleasure. It is focused on feelings and fulfilment, and emphasizes a joyful expression of sexuality and intimacy.

The path to a new awareness includes chapters on:
The Pleasure of Touching
Self-Exploration
Increasing Arousal For Women
Becoming Orgasmic
Learning Control
Overcoming Inhibition

With the current emphasis on the importance of just one sexual partner, this is a timely publication designed to show you just how to make the most of that relationship, and how to build a new sexual partnership.

NON-FICTION/REFERENCE   0 7472 3561 9

Headline Health Kicks

Positive and practical advice to relieve persistent health problems.
Titles available include:

THE PRIME OF YOUR LIFE
Self help during menopause   Pamela Armstrong   £5.99   ☐

STOP COUNTING SHEEP
Self help for insomnia sufferers   Dr Paul Clayton   £5.99   ☐

AM I A MONSTER, OR IS THIS PMS?
Self help for PMS sufferers   Louise Roddon   £5.99   ☐

GET UP AND GO!
Self help for fatigue sufferers   Anne Woodham   £5.99   ☐

You can kick that problem!

All Headline books are available at your local bookshop or newsagent, or can be ordered direct from the publisher. Just tick the titles you want and fill in the form below. Prices and availability subject to change without notice.

Headline Book Publishing Ltd, Cash Sales Department, Bookpoint, 39 Milton Park, Abingdon, OXON, OX14 4TD, UK. If you have a credit card you may order by telephone – 0235 831700.

Please enclose a cheque or postal order made payable to Bookpoint Ltd to the value of the cover price and allow the following for postage and packing:

UK & BFPO: £1.00 for the first book, 50p for the second book and 30p for each additional book ordered up to a maximum charge of £3.00.

OVERSEAS & EIRE: £2.00 for the first book, £1.00 for the second book and 50p for each additional book.

Name...

Address...

....

....

If you would prefer to pay by credit card, please complete:
Please debit my Visa/Access/Diner's Card/American Express (delete as applicable) card no:

Signature..   Expiry date...................